DAREDEVILS AND DAYDREAMERS

DAREDEVILS AND DAYDREAMERS

New Perspectives on Attention-Deficit/ Hyperactivity Disorder

BARBARA D. INGERSOLL, PH.D.

MAIN STREET BOOKS

Doubleday

New York London Toronto Sydney Auckland

A MAIN STREET BOOK

PUBLISHED BY DOUBLEDAY

a division of Bantam Doubleday Dell Publishing Group, Inc.

1540 Broadway, New York, New York 10036

MAIN STREET BOOKS, DOUBLEDAY, and the portrayal of a building with a tree are trademarks of Doubleday, a division of Bantam Doubleday Dell Publishing Group, Inc.

Library of Congress Cataloging-in-Publication Data

Ingersoll, Barbara D., 1945–

Daredevils and daydreamers: new perspectives on attention-deficit/hyperactivity disorder / Barbara D. Ingersoll. — 1st ed.

p.   cm.

Includes bibliographical references and index.

1. Attention-deficit hyperactivity disorder—Popular works.

I. Title.

RJ506.H9I548   1998

616.85′89—dc21   97-22397

                                                       CIP

ISBN 0-385-48757-6

January 1998

First Edition

3   5   7   9   10   8   6   4   2

This book is dedicated to the many committed parents and professionals who, through their unstinting efforts, have done so much to better the lives of individuals with ADHD.

ACKNOWLEDGMENTS

I am grateful to my colleagues, Dr. Harold Eist and Dr. Sam Goldstein, for their careful reading of the manuscript and their many astute comments and suggestions. I owe special thanks to my husband, Tom Ingersoll, for his coordination of a million details, and to my editor, Frances Jones, for her unfailing good cheer and encouragement.

A Personal Note to Readers of This Book

It has been almost exactly ten years since I undertook the task of writing a book for parents of children with Attention-Deficit/Hyperactivity Disorder. When I began work on that book, *Your Hyperactive Child*, I was excited about what Doctors Judith Rapoport and Alan Zametkin subsequently referred to in their foreword as "an explosion of scientific interest in child psychiatry." I was particularly excited, of course, about the burgeoning research on ADHD, and optimistic that this research would form the foundation for better methods of diagnosing and treating a condition that adversely affects so many people.

Even in my excitement and optimism, I didn't dream that we were entering a decade that would bring such dramatic advances in our understanding of ADHD and in our ability to diagnose and treat it. Nor could I have envisioned the profound changes that have taken place for people with ADHD. Parent support groups, for example, were in their infancy a decade ago, and their existence was known only to a handful of people. Now, there is a nationwide network of support groups, the largest of which is CH.A.D.D. (Children and Adults with Attention-Deficit Disorders). This organization, which was founded in Florida in 1987, has grown in less than a decade to 650 chapters, with a membership of more than 36,000.

Thanks in no small part to the efforts of CH.A.D.D. and other support groups, sweeping changes have taken place in the way the needs of youngsters with ADHD are addressed within the school setting. Federal laws, including the Individuals with Disabilities Education Act, the Rehabilitation Act, and the Americans with Disabilities Act, have provided parents with ammunition to take on recalcitrant school systems—and win!

Changes have taken place in the workplace too, as adults with ADHD have begun to insist that their legal rights be upheld. Of course, even the very existence of such large numbers of adults with ADHD was not known ten years ago. Media publicity has enabled many ADHD adults to recognize their symptoms and to obtain treatment for problems that have plagued them for a lifetime.

But this publicity, helpful as it has been, has not always been positive. Some television programs and newspaper articles have portrayed ADHD in an unflattering light, depicting ADHD individuals as crazed and out of control. On occasion, the risks associated with medication have been grossly exaggerated, and some critics have even implied that medication is just the easy way out for lazy parents and teachers.

In the clinical arena, extensive research has confirmed what clinicians have long suspected: among individuals with ADHD, the coexistence of other psychiatric conditions is probably more the rule than the exception, at least among ADHD children, teens, and adults who are referred for treatment. Increased awareness of these comorbid conditions has led to greater diagnostic precision. This, in turn, has resulted in more effective treatments and a better quality of life for people with ADHD.

It has, indeed, been a decade of great change—so much so that, when I began to work on what I thought would be a revised edition of *Your Hyperactive Child,* I soon realized that I faced an impossible task. A revision would not do; so much new information demanded a new book.

This is that book. In preparing it, I have kept some of the material from *Your Hyperactive Child,* material that I believe is still relevant and useful. I've kept some of the examples and vignettes, too, because so many parents have told me that they have seen their children (and themselves) in these pieces.

Because I intend this book to serve as a comprehensive guidebook for parents, teachers, and others in search of information about ADHD, I have made frequent references to the work of many talented scientists and clinicians whose contributions are of potential benefit to individuals with ADHD. Where possible, I have summarized their findings and recommendations as succinctly as I could. However, in some cases I believe that readers would be better served by reading the original work in its entirety, and I have made recommendations accordingly. This, I believe, is a real service at a point in time when books on ADHD have proliferated at a dizzying rate— in itself a good sign and a portent of more good things to come.

—*Barbara D. Ingersoll, Ph.D.*

CONTENTS

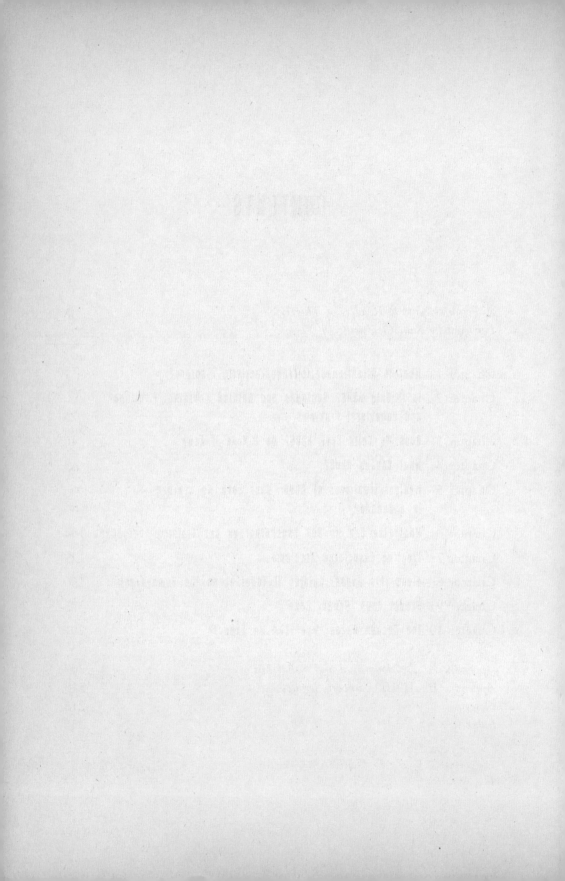

FOREWORD

by Samuel Goldstein, Ph.D.

As we prepare to enter the twenty-first century, the scientific advances of the past decade place us on the threshold of a limitless future, one few of us can imagine. At no time in history have there been so many—and such rapid—advances in science, technology, medicine, and education.

Over the past decade, Attention Deficit/Hyperactivity Disorder (ADHD) has become the most widely researched topic in child development and the mental health issue most often cited in the lay press. New ground is broken daily and our knowledge about ADHD grows at an exponential rate. We have increasingly come to recognize that, as Dr. Michael Rutter points out, nature and nurture do not operate independently of each other, but are complexly intertwined to produce human behavior.*

With the publication of her first text on this subject in 1988, *Your Hyperactive Child: A Parent's Guide to Coping with Attention Deficit Disorder,* Barbara Ingersoll offered a reasoned and reasonable approach to assist parents to understand, but most importantly, help children with ADHD. Her ground-breaking text was followed by dozens of publications by authors worldwide, myself included.† Many have emulated her approach and model. It is not surprising that her original text has been one of the bestselling volumes on this subject for both parents and professionals.

In her current book, Dr. Ingersoll brings to a close a decade of rapid

---

* Rutter, M. L. "Nature-nurture integration: The example of antisocial behavior." *American Psychologist,* 52, 1997, 390-398.

† Goldstein, S. and M. Goldstein. *Hyperactivity: Why Won't My Child Pay Attention?* New York, NY: Wiley, 1992.

growth and understanding in the field of ADHD, and positions parents at the threshold of the twenty-first century. Dr. Ingersoll deftly and in a very practical, understandable format, summarizes the enormous research literature on ADHD and provides parents with workable guidelines to assist them in dealing with the ADHD child—beginning with the diagnostic process and moving through intervention and help for co-occurring problems. As ADHD represents a problem that must be managed rather than cured, Dr. Ingersoll's supportive approach provides parents with hope, motivation, and the tools necessary to help their children. This is particularly important. An increasing body of research on children's ability to cope with adversity finds that positive parental relationships are essential. Parents' ability to be proud, patient, and persistent when advocating for their children is likely to be among the best predictors of positive adult outcome for everyone.* This is not to suggest that parents should feel guilty if their children are struggling but rather that they understand and accept the responsibility they have for structuring their children's lives in ways that protect and insulate not just children with ADHD but all children.

The United Nations Convention on the Rights of the Child† has advocated that as an international community, it is the duty of each citizen of all nations to ensure that children's rights to survival, protection, development, and education are fulfilled. Our emphasis upon the best interests of all children, their rights and dignity, represents a bright star as we pass into the twenty-first century. As a society we must understand and deal effectively with the alarming trend of problems among our youth. For parents and professionals working with children with ADHD, this future trend offers great hope. It is this critical hope and goal for children with ADHD that *Daredevils and Daydreamers* addresses. This text first and foremost respects the rights of the child, while supporting the needs of the family. It is a text that does, as did Dr. Ingersoll's original work, make a significant contribution to the field and to the best interests of all children. For in the end, no matter how effective and efficient our

---

* Katz, M. *On Playing a Poor Hand Well*. Chicago, IL: Norton, 1997.

† Limber, S.P. & M. G. Flekkoy. "The UN convention on the rights of the child: It's relevance for social scientists." *Social Policy Report: Society for Research and Child Development,* **IX(2),**1995.

treatments are for Attention Deficit/Hyperactivity Disorder, it is the course of society and the outcome for all children that will best predict and contribute to our success in the treatment of ADHD.

—*Sam Goldstein, Ph.D.*

Neurology, Learning and Behavior Center
University of Utah

CHAPTER 1

WHAT IS ATTENTION-DEFICIT/HYPERACTIVITY DISORDER?

Overview: Then and Now

Then: Ten years ago, most people still thought of ADHD as a condition that affected children only. And, although some researchers had already told us that ADHD children could have attentional problems without hyperactivity, ADHD children were usually depicted as whirling dervishes who careened through life, leaving a swath of destruction in their wake.

Now: We now know that there is a sizable subgroup of quiet daydreamers whose inability to organize themselves and focus on the task at hand makes it impossible for them to meet the demands of everyday life. As we've learned more about ADHD in its many manifestations, diagnostic guidelines have also changed.

We know, too, that many children with ADHD continue to have symptoms as adults. Again, there were hints of this ten years ago, but our knowledge of ADHD in adults has grown exponentially. In fact, increased awareness of the problems of adults with ADHD is one of the most significant advances in the past decade.

The past decade has also launched us into the age of e-mail, the Web, and the Internet. There are now many home pages devoted to ADHD, and people who have an interest in ADHD find it increasingly easy to keep abreast of new developments in the field. But increased media publicity about ADHD, while often informative, has sometimes contributed more confusion than clarification. In a spate of television shows, books, and magazine articles, ADHD has come under attack as an invented disorder, and parents have been made to feel guilty for giving stimulant medication to their children.

Who Is the Child with ADHD?

When she entered the pediatrician's office with four-year-old Timmy in tow, Mrs. Evans burst out: "Doctor, you've got to do something!" Glancing at her son, she went on. "I don't feel good about asking you to put Timmy on Ritalin—in fact, I hate the idea—but Timmy is making me crazy. He's on the go every waking minute. He's broken every toy he's ever owned and our house looks like a disaster area. We've tried to childproof the house, but nothing is safe from him. Last week I caught him with a pair of garden shears, getting ready to give the dog a haircut.

He's not a mean child; he's really got a heart of gold, but the other kids avoid him because he's so rough. In fact, I don't think that his preschool will take him back next year because he's such a handful. If we don't do something soon, I just don't know what's going to happen to him—or to me!"

From the bleachers, Jeremy's parents watched in dismay as he threw his bat to the ground and stormed off the field in tears when he struck out. It was an all-too-familiar scene, not only to Jeremy's parents, but to his teammates and his Little League coach as well. As long as things were going his way, Jeremy was fine. But let something go wrong—something like striking out or a bad call from an umpire—and Jeremy simply fell apart, wailing, cursing, and throwing himself on the ground.

His teachers, too, knew that Jeremy had a short fuse. Although he excelled in academics and was generally an enthusiastic student, Jeremy had difficulty when classmates didn't agree with his ideas. On the playground, he was likely to erupt in shrieks and tantrums if a playmate teased him or flouted the rules in a game. Sadly, some of Jeremy's peers found these outbursts amusing and had begun to make a game of provoking him.

Fourteen-year-old Elizabeth, a pretty girl with beautiful brown eyes and curly hair, sat quietly between her parents in the guidance counselor's office. The counselor looked up from a sheaf of papers in her hand and shook her head slowly, as if puzzled. "Liz, you know we all want to help you—that's why we're here today. But just listen to these reports from your teachers." Glancing at the papers in her hand, she read the comments: "Bright, but not working to her potential . . . Often seems to be in another world . . . Six out of ten lab reports missing . . . Rough draft of "Seasons" paper was due two weeks ago: where is it? . . . Seldom remembers to bring her instrument for band practice . . . Never has PE clothes."

"Liz," the counselor continued, "I don't know what to suggest. You're too old to have someone follow you around to remind you of things you have to do. Everyone knows you can do the work, but your teachers aren't willing to be baby-sitters. They're starting to wonder if Hartwell is really the right school for you or if you'd be happier someplace else."

What is attention-deficit/hyperactivity disorder? As you can see, ADHD has many faces, so identifying and diagnosing ADHD children can be confusing. The confusion has been compounded by the many terms used over the years to describe the condition—terms like "minimal brain damage," "minimal brain dysfunction," "hyperkinesis," "hyperactivity," and, most recently, "attention-deficit/hyperactivity disorder (ADHD). These changes in terminology reflect changes in our thinking about the nature, the cause, and the course of the disorder itself. As a child psychologist who has worked with ADHD children and their families for over twenty-five years, I have lived through many of these changes.

I recall, for example, the belief in the fifties and sixties that inattentive, impulsive, hyperactive children suffered from brain damage. Since medical tests could not actually identify the presumed damage, the term "minimal brain dysfunction" (MBD) was coined to describe these children. Experts recommended classrooms designed to avoid distracting these youngsters. Windows of frosted glass, bare bulletin boards, and teachers dressed in drab colors and wearing no makeup were suggested. How these suggestions could be put in place in the local schools was never clear and, to my knowledge, no one ever found out whether the approach was really effective.

By the mid-sixties, stimulant medication was increasingly used to treat hyperactive youngsters and there was an upsurge of research into the nature and treatment of the disorder. Scientists focused on excessive motor activity as the core of the problem and the terms "hyperkinesis" and "hyperactivity" replaced the term MBD. Through the mid-seventies, gadget-loving researchers happily availed themselves of all kinds of equipment designed to assess activity, from activity meters worn on wrists or ankles to—picture this—a "stabilometric cushion" that counted how many times a youngster bounced in place without leaving his chair.

In the seventies, researchers began to focus on problems with attention span in ADHD children. The work of psychologist Virginia Douglas at McGill University suggested that the problems of hyperactive children had less to do with excessive activity than with a short attention span and impulsivity that made them unable to "stop, look, and listen" before acting. The name of the syndrome was officially changed to attention deficit disorder by the American Psychiatric Association and researchers put aside their activity monitors in favor of tests designed to measure attention and concentration.

Most recently, the American Psychiatric Association has renamed the syndrome attention-deficit/hyperactivity disorder, or ADHD. They have spelled out diagnostic criteria, discussed in detail below.

Diagnostic Guidelines

How can we tell the difference between a youngster who is just bouncy and exuberant and one who is truly hyperactive? What about the child who daydreams in class or doodles while the lesson goes unheeded? What should we make of a disorganized, forgetful, absentminded youngster who is always out of step with those around him? Do all of these children have ADHD?

Guidelines for diagnosing ADHD are outlined in the *Diagnostic and Statistical Manual of Mental Disorders,* Fourth Edition (DSM-IV), published by the American Psychiatric Association.[1] These guidelines aren't perfect, but they do provide a common language and a set of common standards that professionals can use to make a diagnosis.

In DSM-IV, the diverse symptoms of ADHD are grouped into two categories, *inattention* and *hyperactivity-impulsivity.* In order to be diagnosed with ADHD, a child must have at least six symptoms of inattention *or* six symptoms of hyperactivity-impulsivity, as described below.

The DSM-IV also stipulates that symptoms must be present before the age of seven and that they must persist for at least six months. Symptoms must also pose problems in two or more settings and there must be "significant impairment in social, academic, or occupational functioning."

Inattention

■ **Often fails to give close attention to details or makes careless mistakes in schoolwork, work, or other activities.** The ADHD child is usually in such a rush to complete his schoolwork that the final product is messy and filled with errors. "Proofreading" and "editing" might just as well be words in a foreign language as far as many ADHD students are concerned, and a request to recopy a paper is likely to be met with howls of protest.

At home, chores are done in slapdash fashion: when setting the table, the ADHD child may remember knives and spoons but forget forks. He may put out glasses but no plates, salt but no pepper, and butter but no bread. When it's his turn to clear the table, perhaps half of the dirty dishes will make it as far as the kitchen; none, however, will actually be put in the dishwasher.

■ **Often has difficulty sustaining attention in tasks or play activities.** Although people with ADHD are at their worst when they have to concentrate on monotonous tasks, some ADHD youngsters have difficulty paying attention even when they are engaged in activities they enjoy. It's not uncommon for an ADHD child to change activities so many times in a day that by evening, the playroom is littered with toys from one end to the other. It's not uncommon, either, to see a Little Leaguer with ADHD standing out in right field—where else would a coach place him?—lost in contemplation of the clouds overhead or the dandelions at his feet, oblivious of the game going on around him.

■ **Often does not seem to listen when spoken to directly.** Many parents of ADHD children report having had their child's hearing checked at an early age because the child never seemed to hear them when they called or told him to do something. Older children and adults with ADHD often seem to be "in another world" when they are engrossed in watching television or reading the newspaper. It's not that ADHD people can never pay attention: rather, they have difficulty in regulating attention—keeping it focused when necessary and changing the focus when that becomes necessary. Thus, transitions may be hard for ADHD people, especially if they are asked to stop an interesting or enjoyable activity to go on to something else.

■ **Often does not follow through on instructions and fails to finish schoolwork, chores, or duties in the workplace.** As parents of ADHD children can attest, it is futile to give these children multiple-step directions. Told to go upstairs, wash his face and hands, and bring down his math book, the typical ADHD child may get as far as the top of the stairs, become distracted, and engage in another activity until an angry parent yells up to remind him of the purpose of the trip.

People with ADHD tend to be enthusiastic at the start of a task, but their enthusiasm wanes as the task goes on. The parents of one such child, surveying several unfinished model planes, three Scout projects abandoned in various stages of completion, and a stack of incomplete thank-you notes for birthday gifts received six months earlier, ruefully described the youngster as "The King of Unfinished Projects."

■ **Often has difficulty organizing tasks and activities.** It is difficult for people with ADHD to set priorities, plan ahead, and proceed in a methodical way. When an ADHD child is faced with the task of cleaning his room, for example, he might be so overwhelmed with the task of imposing order on chaos that he simply wads up everything in sight and stuffs it under the bed.

School places particular demands on youngsters to be well organized, but, for many "organizationally challenged" ADHD youngsters, these demands are impossible to meet. Some bright, hardworking ADHD youngsters earn failing grades in school because they are too disorganized and forgetful to turn in their completed homework and projects. Others are so scattered that they forget to write down the homework assignment or take the appropriate books home, so they can't even start the work, much less complete it.

■ **Often avoids, dislikes, or is reluctant to engage in tasks that require sustained mental effort (such as schoolwork or homework).** People with ADHD are at their worst with boring or repetitive tasks. Unfortunately, this describes many of the tasks assigned in school, so the same child who can spend hours engrossed in sorting his baseball cards must be repeatedly called back to task in the classroom. And since few ADHD youngsters can face the tedium of homework after a long day in school, battles over homework are waged from the elementary years all the way through high school.

As adults, ADHD individuals continue to abhor the tedium of paperwork. Asked to complete a multipage form, for example, they may get as far as the first page, then put the whole thing aside until later. But "later" never comes, as I can attest from all of the half-completed forms that are returned to me by parents of the ADHD youngsters I see in my practice.

■ **Often loses things necessary for tasks or activities (e.g., toys, school assignments, pencils, books, or tools).** We all occasionally misplace our keys or glasses, but, for the child with ADHD, these are daily occurrences—much to the chagrin of parents who bear the cost of replacing lost items. Again, I know this from firsthand experience: the toys, clothes, books, glasses, and umbrellas left in my waiting room over the years would provide the merchandise for a truly mammoth yard sale. And since ADHD tends to run in families, I'm not surprised when a parent calls an hour before the first appointment to say that he or she has lost the directions to my office. I'm not surprised, either, when that same parent arrives without paperwork for the appointment, having left it behind on the kitchen counter.

■ **Is often easily distracted by extraneous stimuli.** Even when the task is important, the ADHD youngster can be lured away by something as inconsequential as the cat walking across the room. This is the child who, when sent upstairs to dress, can be found in his room five minutes before the school bus arrives, naked except for one sock, playing happily with the gerbil. This same youngster, as an adult, might decide to change the oil in the car ten minutes before dinner guests arrive because a trip to the garage to get the grill reminded him that the car was due for an oil change.

It is not just external events that can distract the ADHD individual; indeed, many are so distracted by their own thoughts that their conversation is disjointed and hard to follow. Asking an ADHD youngster to explain the rules of a game or describe the plot of a movie is usually an exercise in futility, since the resulting explanation may be incomprehensible even to someone who is familiar with the game or has seen the movie.

- **Is often forgetful in daily activities.** People with ADHD always seem to be "a day late and a dollar short." They miss important deadlines, forget appointments, and are never where they are supposed to be when they are supposed to be there. As they enter their teens and adult years, they may be considered rude and inconsiderate when they leave friends waiting for them at the theater or the dinner table and when they forget birthdays, anniversaries, and other important events.

Hyperactivity-Impulsivity

- **Often fidgets with hands or feet or squirms in seat.** Even when an ADHD youngster is engrossed in an exciting movie or game, some part of his body may be in constant motion. This fidgetiness can be costly and annoying, since it may take the form of chewing on clothing, picking at upholstery or wallpaper, and doodling on inappropriate surfaces. Some ADHD adults learn to compensate by keeping their hands busy with needlework or knitting. Without such an outlet, many simply drum their fingers, bite their nails, or jiggle their feet when they are confined to a seated position.

- **Often leaves seat in classroom or in other situations in which remaining seated is expected.** Teenagers and adults with ADHD are less likely than younger ADHD individuals to dart about in an excessively active fashion, but many find it difficult to remain still. As adults, they may turn this need for constant movement to good advantage, as in the case of a busy dentist or emergency room physician who dashes from cubicle to cubicle, attending to various patients. Others find success in the world of sales, where they can move about all day, or in other fields that require high energy and lots of activity.

ADHD children, however, are confined by the constraints of the classroom. Sometimes an understanding teacher will allow them to stand while doing their work or send them on errands around the building, but, for the most part, they are constantly chided for their inability to remain quietly in place.

- **Often runs about or climbs excessively in situations in which it is inappropriate (in adolescents or adults, may be limited to subjective feelings of restlessness).** As noted authority Dr. Paul Wender said of these youngsters, "Parents frequently report that after an active and restless infancy the child stood and walked at an early age and then, like an infant King Kong, burst the bars of his crib and marched forth to destroy the house."

ADHD children seem driven to explore as much of the world around them as they can reach, even at risk to life and limb. Some are drawn to danger like a magnet, and their parents recount tales of two-year-olds who turn on stoves and climb out third-story windows. In fact, ADHD children are much more likely than other children to experience several serious accidents during childhood and many are familiar faces in the emergency room at their local hospital.

- **Often has difficulty playing or engaging in leisure activities quietly.** People with ADHD annoy others by incessant humming, whistling, singing, chanting, and making strange and unusual noises. It's common for children playing with toy cars or planes to accompany their play with loud sound effects: the ADHD child, however, may make just as much noise while drawing a picture, working on a jigsaw puzzle, or playing with Legos.

- **Is often "on the go" or often acts as if "driven by a motor."** People who don't have ADHD can become exhausted by the frenetic pace set by someone with ADHD. This was brought home to me when we were invited to the beach house of delightful friends, both of whom have ADHD, as do their children. Their warm hospitality was a treat— for the first day. By the second day, my energy began to flag as we moved from the tennis courts to the golf course to the beach and then to dinner and then on to a pub to listen to Irish folk music into the wee hours. By the third day, they were all still going strong ("Come on, let's hit the boardwalk") but I was ready to be taken home by ambulance!

■ **Often blurts out answers before questions have been completed.** Because the ADHD child guesses at directions rather than listening carefully, he may go charging off in the wrong direction, not realizing his error until it is too late. In the classroom, he blurts out answers and offers unsolicited comments. On the rare occasions when he does remember to raise his hand before speaking, his gestures are so frantic and accompanied by such spectacular sound effects that the teacher must either call on him or call him down for his antics.

People with ADHD blurt out in other ways too. Having heard part of a conversation, they may jump in with a completely off-topic remark. They may make tactless comments ("Gosh, what an ugly baby!"), ask inappropriate questions ("How much did that necklace cost you?"), or commit other social gaffes which cause others to consider them rude and boorish.

■ **Often has difficulty awaiting turn.** Standing in line is torture for ADHD children. Waiting for anything, in fact, is painful. In restaurants—even fast-food restaurants—they writhe with impatience until the food arrives. Then, having eaten, they can't wait quietly until others have finished: instead, they begin to torment their siblings, make obnoxious noises with their soft drinks, climb about under the table, and just generally annoy the daylights out of their dining companions.

I find it instructive to play Candyland with young ADHD patients. Some are so impatient that they begin playing the game before the board has been set up. While others are able to delay long enough to help arrange the board and even to politely urge me to go first, it is only a matter of minutes before the child, under the guise of "helping," begins to select my cards for me. Then the child, again being helpful, moves my marker after selecting and interpreting the card. Soon I can sit back and observe as the child plays the game without me.

■ **Often interrupts or intrudes on others (e.g. butts into conversations or games).** ADHD children seldom stop to survey a situation before they barge in. Other children might observe from the sidelines and even ask permission before venturing to join an ongoing game or activity. Not so the ADHD child; if it looks like fun, in he goes without a moment's hesitation. And the fact that Mom is in the bathroom or on the telephone doesn't deter him when he wants Mom's attention.

Beyond the Diagnostic Guidelines

Although the diagnostic guidelines in DSM-IV are helpful, they are not perfect. As long ago as 1981, Dr. Russell Barkley criticized the guidelines on the grounds that impulsivity, hyperactivity, and attentional problems are *not* the only major symptoms in many ADHD individuals.[2] Instead, he pointed out, his research and that of others demonstrated that ADHD children have significant difficulty following rules: even when they know the rules, they seem to lack the self-control to adhere to them except under very close supervision. Thus, he argued, *deficits in rule-governed behavior* should be considered the central problem in ADHD.

Dr. Barkley has since modified his theory to focus on impulsivity as the core problem in ADHD.[3] Specifically, he believes that the problems of ADHD individuals stem from their inability to pause or delay before they react. According to Dr. Barkley, this deficit might explain the entire range of ADHD behavior, including poor learning from past experience, difficulty abiding by rules, and lowered mindfulness of future consequences and events.

Is Dr. Barkley's theory correct? In science, one cannot "prove" a theory. Instead, a theory is considered helpful if it can account for what we know about the condition under study and if it helps to guide research and thereby advance our knowledge. Dr. Barkley's theory does appear to account for much of what we know about ADHD, and it has served to generate and guide research on ADHD.

From Toddler to Teenager and Beyond: ADHD Across the Life Span

As children grow and change, so do the problems associated with ADHD. Over time, the hyperactive youngster's level of activity diminishes. Over time, too, the disorganized daydreamer may learn ways to compensate for lapses in attention. Even so, the amount of energy invested in compensating for problems with attention and organization takes a heavy toll.

Infancy

Mothers of many ADHD children report high levels of activity from the earliest days—sometimes, in fact, even while the child is still in the womb. Hyperactive infants are often restless and difficult to hold, so feedings and diaper changes can be a challenge. It may be a challenge, too, to keep a hyperactive youngster in his crib, since many are accomplished escape artists. Parents may resort to such extreme measures as using chicken wire to make a crib escapeproof, lest the child injure himself when he climbs out.

"Sammy's been a pistol from the minute he was born. The doctor didn't even have to give him a smack on the butt to get him started: he let out with a yell and hasn't quit since then. Take your eyes off him for a minute and he'll find something to get into. He can crawl faster than most people can run and he can climb like a little monkey, so nothing is safe from him."

In looking back, you might not describe your child as having been excessively active. You might even remember the early years as a calm, happy period, especially if your child has a pleasant temperament. Chances are, however, that you can recall early and repeated bouts of sickness: ADHD children are particularly prone to colds, upper respiratory infections, and ear infections, perhaps as a result of problems with the immune system (see Chapter 4). You also might have noticed some delays in language development, since some ADHD children are late in beginning to talk.

The Preschool Years

Excessive activity continues to characterize many ADHD children during the preschool years. Even parents who don't have to contend with constant running, bouncing, and jumping may be worn out by a busy youngster who gets into things as soon as their backs are turned. Taking such a child to stores and other public places can be a traumatic experience, since even older youngsters with ADHD seem compelled to touch and handle everything they see. Because these youngsters are inclined to dart away in crowded malls and dash out into busy parking lots, desperate parents may resort to using a harness to control the child. (Thankfully, some genius—probably the parent of an ADHD child—came up with Velcro "handcuffs" which link parent and child together without drawing disapproving looks from other people.)

"Joshua is a sweetheart. But it's murder to take him anyplace because he wants to get into everything he sees and he can take off like a bullet if you turn your back."

Toilet training the ADHD toddler can also be a struggle, since many continue to have bowel and bladder accidents well past the age at which most other children are completely trained. Often the youngster is delayed in other ways, too, such as in the fine-motor skills required for many preschool cut-and-paste projects. Speech and language delays are also surprisingly common, as we discuss in Chapter 2.

If an ADHD child is prone to aggressive outbursts, his welcome in play groups may be short-lived. Other parents are understandably perturbed by the presence of a youngster who impulsively pushes, shoves, hits, and grabs toys from the children around him. Day-care providers quickly lose patience with a child who refuses to settle at naptime and who must be physically hauled back inside, kicking and screaming in protest, when outdoor playtime ends.

Middle Childhood

Because school presents such demands for self-control, even ADHD children who can squeak by in other settings may fail miserably in elementary school, where they are expected to follow instructions, work independently, and abide by classroom rules. The ADHD child, with his restlessness and short attention span, is quickly labeled "immature" or "uncooperative." This view is reinforced by the fact that the child is often disorganized, forgetful, and messy—qualities abhorred by most teachers. If the child is also loud, boisterous, and prone to getting into wrangles on the playground, a teacher's patience may be strained to the breaking point.

Learning difficulties and disabilities, common in ADHD children, further complicate the child's situation in school. As we shall see in Chapter 2, even bright ADHD children may not perform well in school.

At home, parents grow increasingly impatient with a child who just can't seem to do what is expected. Mornings are chaotic as parents try to hurry their "morning dawdler" out the door before the school bus departs, and evenings are filled with screaming matches over chores and homework.

Many ADHD children also have great difficulty making and keeping friends. Some, in fact, are "social outcasts" who are actively rejected by other children; others are simply ignored by their peers and left to go their way alone.

Adolescence

Only a minority of ADHD children—perhaps fifteen percent or so—are symptom free when they enter their teen years.[4] Now, of course, the young person is faced with the challenges and changes that adolescence brings. Combined with the baggage he already carries, the ADHD teenager can face a trying and demoralizing time indeed.

School performance in particular is apt to be a problem for the ADHD adolescent. Even very bright youngsters who are able to compensate for their attentional problems in elementary school may fall apart when faced with the demands of middle school. Grades drop precipitously and failure becomes increasingly common. In high school, parents escalate from worried to frantic as college admission looms closer. "How will he ever get into a decent college?" they ask. "And how's he going to make a living without a college education?"

Other fears confront parents of ADHD teenagers whose chronic problems with rules have made chaos of family life and even brought them into conflict with the law. As one parent put it, "I used to worry that he wouldn't get into college. Now I just hope that he stays out of jail."

The Adult Years

Thanks to the work of such pioneers as Dr. Paul Wender at the University of Utah and to the more recent work of others such as Dr. Joseph Biederman at Harvard and Dr. Kevin Murphy at the University of Massachusetts, we know much more about ADHD adults than we did a decade ago. We know, for example, that although the most obvious symptoms of ADHD may appear to decrease in intensity with increasing age, problems with attention and organization persist.

In adults, emotional overreactivity, rapid mood changes, and impulsivity are common symptoms. Brief but explosive temper outbursts can put a serious strain on personal relationships, although many ADHD adults have difficulty understanding the effect such outbursts have on others. ADHD adults also complain that they can't handle the stresses of daily life, and many find it difficult to sit down and relax. On the positive side, some channel excess energy into hobbies, home improvement projects, volunteer work, and overtime at work. On the negative side, their need for movement, stimulation, and change can be a vast source of annoyance to roommates, spouses, and coworkers.

Prognosis

Lurking in the mind of every parent of an ADHD child is the gnawing worry about how the child will fare as an adult. Many parents have told me: "I can live with the day-to-day hassles, but it's when I think about his future that I get really worried. What's going to happen to him when he's an adult?"

What does happen to ADHD youngsters when they become adults? Certainly, the statistics are enough to frighten parents of ADHD children right out of their socks. For example, the research of Dr. Russell Barkley at the University of Massachusetts indicates that impulsive, risk-taking youngsters continue to take risks as teenagers and adults, but the stakes get higher as the youngsters get older.[5] Dr. Barkley has found that as teenagers and young adults, ADHD individuals take risks with their health by neglecting diet and exercise and by engaging in such unhealthy behaviors as smoking and drinking. They take risks in other ways too: young ADHD drivers, especially those who have coexisting conduct or oppositional disorders, tend to be somewhat reckless and erratic behind the wheel.[6] And while they don't seem to be more sexually active than others their age, ADHD young adults aren't careful about practicing safe sex, so they have more sexually transmitted diseases. They also tend to have children at an early age, unlike their age mates, who wait until their twenties or thirties to bear children.

Some ADHD adolescents also violate rules and the rights of others, a pattern known as conduct disorder (see Chapter 2). In conduct-disordered adolescents who commit serious offenses, antisocial tendencies often persist and become chronic in adult life. There is research that suggests an unusually high rate of conduct disorder in ADHD children: Dr. Barkley, for example, found that almost half of a group of ADHD adolescents seen at his clinic during childhood could be diagnosed with conduct disorder at follow-up eight years later.[7]

Bear in mind, however, that at least some of these findings are based on *clinical samples* rather than on groups of ADHD children drawn from the general population, so they might not reflect what happens to ADHD children in general. In the past, clinical samples often consisted of only the most difficult, treatment-resistant ADHD youngsters.* To help you understand this, let's look at the process through which an ADHD child might become part of a clinical sample.

- Step 1. Parents and/or teachers become concerned about the child's inattentiveness, hyperactivity, impulsivity, or other symptoms associated with ADHD.
- Step 2. The school provides appropriate services (accommodations, assessment, behavior management program) and/or the parent seeks help from a pediatrician, who then prescribes stimulant medication. If these interventions are *not* effective, the child moves to Step 3.

---

* More current researchers have recognized the problems involved in using clinical samples. In fact, in the large-scale NIMH Multisite Multimodal Treatment Study of Children with ADHD now in progress, specific efforts were made to generate a representative sample of children with ADHD.

■ Step 3. The child is referred to a mental health professional who provides treatment involving some combination of therapy, parent counseling, behavior management, and medication. If these interventions are *not* effective, the child moves to Step 4.

■ Step 4. The child is placed in a special education setting and/or referred to a local mental health professional who specializes in treating ADHD. If these interventions are *not* effective, the child moves to Step 5.

■ Step 5. The child is placed in residential care or is referred to a specialty clinic headed by a nationally known expert in ADHD. If the latter is the case, the child will probably become part of the expert's pool of research subjects from which the researcher will draw conclusions about ADHD children in general.

The problem with drawing conclusions based on the sample of children who have reached Step 5 is obvious: researchers see only those children for whom all other treatments have failed. They—and we—have no way of knowing what happens to the ADHD children who don't make it past Steps 2, 3, or 4. There are no outcome studies of these children, but logic and my own clinical experience suggest that for many, the future bodes as well for them as for youngsters without ADHD.

Critical Factors for Adult Success. Bearing all of the above in mind, there are some predictions we can make about outcome for ADHD children. We know, for example, that factors such as intelligence, family functioning, and family socioeconomic status are related to outcome.

As common sense would dictate, ADHD children have the greatest likelihood of success when they are raised in intact families with the financial and emotional resources to provide for their needs. Intelligence, too, plays a part: bright ADHD youngsters have an advantage over less well-endowed children.

ADHD children who are least likely to be successful as adults are those who come from impoverished families who hold academic achievement in low regard and in which strife and even violence are common. If antisocial and aggressive behavior characterize the family and the child, so much the worse: the most important factor associated with adult antisocial behavior is a history of aggressive and antisocial behavior in the child and his family.

Good child-rearing practices clearly play an important role in outcome. Parents who are neglectful or who vacillate between excessively tolerant and excessively harsh responses to behavior can expect problems with their children, especially those children who have ADHD.

Comorbidity, the coexistence of other psychiatric and behavioral problems, plays a role too. ADHD children who have coexisting problems are more difficult to treat and have less likelihood of successful outcome, as discussed in Chapter 2.

How Widespread Is the Problem?

It is generally agreed that ADHD affects at least three to five percent of children in this country. However, figures can vary dramatically, depending on how stringently diagnostic criteria are applied.

Gender Differences. Boys are still diagnosed at a higher rate than girls, although the gap has narrowed in a decade from six or seven boys for every girl to about four or five boys per girl. This change probably reflects better "case finding" over the years, since researchers suggested that many ADHD girls are overlooked because their problems are less visible and less annoying to adults than the problems of ADHD boys.

The fact that boys are still diagnosed with ADHD much more frequently than girls may mean that scales designed to identify ADHD boys do not detect girls with ADHD. In fact, when separate norms are used for boys and girls, ADHD shows up equally as often in girls as in boys.[8] And when adolescents rate their own problems with attention, males and females report problems with equal frequency.[9]

Cross-cultural Findings. What about the incidence of ADHD in other countries? ADHD has always been diagnosed much more frequently in the United States than in other countries. Does this reflect differences in national character—our genetic inheritance from restless, risk-taking ancestors who braved the stormy waters of the Atlantic to conquer a new world? This is a romantic picture, and one in which there might even be a grain of truth. But, in fact, it is probably differences in diagnostic practices more than anything else that accounts for the greater frequency with which ADHD is diagnosed in the United States compared with other countries.

In Italy, for example, the diagnosis of ADHD is virtually never made and stimulant medications are not available. Does this mean that ADHD doesn't exist in Italy? Not really. When similar diagnostic criteria are used, rates of ADHD appear similar across countries, including Italy.[10] The difference lies in the fact that Americans tend to see ADHD symptoms as the result of biological and organic factors. Italian psychiatrists, however, like psychiatrists in many other Western European countries, are more likely to view these behavior patterns as the result of social and psychological factors ("His parents are rigid and demanding"). Thus, many children who would be diagnosed with ADHD in the United States are not so diagnosed in Italy.

Is ADHD Just Another Fad?

In the past several years ADHD has been showcased on television talk shows and quasi-news programs, in newspaper articles, and in popular magazines. This publicity has heightened awareness about ADHD among parents, educators, and health professionals. Parents who have seen their children's difficulties depicted in a television program often acted on this information to obtain an evaluation of their child's problems. Many, too, have seen themselves, a spouse, or a close friend in programs and articles about adult ADHD and have taken similar action.

But not all media coverage has been positive: some critics have charged that ADHD is nothing more than the latest fad. Others have suggested that children diagnosed with ADHD are victims of a conspiracy involving doctors, drug companies, and parents and teachers who want to drug perfectly normal children for their own selfish reasons.

To those of us who live and work with ADHD children, these are fighting words. Parents, teachers, and mental health professionals know that ADHD is real, and so are the problems of children and adults who suffer from ADHD. But in our zeal to identify and help individuals with ADHD, have we become too quick to diagnose ADHD? Do we, as the critics charge, sometimes see ADHD in every active five-year-old and in every adolescent who is bored in school?

It is true that so many more children are diagnosed with ADHD now than in the past. In fact, Dr. James Swanson's group at the University of

California at Irvine reported that the number of people diagnosed with ADHD in the U.S. actually doubled between 1990 and 1993.[11] Why? Have we gone overboard with this diagnosis? Or are we just *better at recognizing and diagnosing* ADHD? Could it be that our *lifestyle* has changed so that these youngsters have a more difficult time fitting in?

I do *not* believe that we are overdiagnosing ADHD. Instead, I think that the reason we have identified so many ADHD individuals in recent years probably reflects a combination of several factors, as follows:

■ **Heightened Awareness of ADHD:** Years ago, children who couldn't sit still, pay attention, or follow rules were just considered "bad" or "spoiled" or "lazy." As Dr. Sam Goldstein and I observed in *Attention Deficit Disorder and Learning Disabilities,* children who failed in school were labeled "slow," or "mentally retarded." Some succeeded in spite of the odds, but many others were warehoused in special education programs or juvenile detention facilities. Others dropped out of school and entered the workforce as manual laborers or eked out a marginal existence on the fringes of society.

Parents today, however, are not willing to let their children be written off in such cavalier fashion. Thanks to the parent-support-group movement, which began in the sixties with parents of mentally retarded youngsters, parents have learned that there is strength in numbers. Under the banner of groups such as CH.A.D.D. (Children and Adults with Attention Deficit Disorders) and ADDA (Attention Deficit Disorder Association), parents have united with concerned professionals to advocate. successfully for the rights of ADHD individuals in the public schools and in the workplace.

■ **Improved Diagnostic Practices:** It wasn't that long ago that psychiatry was dominated by the notion that disturbances in behavior were caused by disturbances within the *mind*. In the past few decades, the focus has shifted to disturbances within the *brain* as the source of disordered behavior and emotions. In the process, our approach to diagnosing psychiatric conditions has moved toward increased precision. No longer, for example, does a pediatrician make a diagnosis of ADHD based solely on the child's behavior in the office—a good thing, too, since as many as eighty percent of ADHD children do not display obvious signs of ADHD in the doctor's office. No doubt many such youngsters went undiagnosed in the past.

Increased diagnostic precision has also revealed the extent to which ADHD coexists with other learning and behavior problems. In fact, recent research has clearly shown that the coexistence of one or more additional conditions with ADHD is more often the rule than the exception, as we discuss in Chapter 2. In the past, however, a youngster with prominent symptoms of anxiety or depression might be diagnosed only with an anxiety disorder or a mood disorder, while the associated ADHD went undetected.

Now, of course, we know that the diagnosis of ADHD is often not an either-or proposition. Thus, troubled youngsters in whom ADHD was previously overlooked are now also being diagnosed with ADHD. (Interestingly, epidemiological studies indicate that the prevalence of psychiatric disorders such as mood and anxiety disorders is increasing in our population, especially among children and adolescents, so this may further swell the ranks of this group.)

Another group overlooked in the past consists of adults with ADHD. Their number in the population has been conservatively estimated at between two and five million[12] and, in increasing numbers they are seeking treatment for ADHD. When these adults are successfully treated, they are quick to spot the symptoms in others—family members, friends, and coworkers—and to pass the word along that help is available.

▪ **Social Changes:** Looking back a few centuries or so, we can see how people with ADHD might have fared better under different social conditions. The same qualities that cause an ADHD child so much difficulty in contemporary society—boundless energy, a need for novelty, hair-trigger responses—might have served a person well in the primeval savannah, on the battlefield, or on the American frontier.

But we don't have to go that far back in time to note dramatic changes in the way people live. A generation ago, children had much more freedom than children growing up today. Back then, Saturdays were spent riding bikes, exploring the woods and fields, building forts, and catching wiggly things in the creek. Children returned late in the day, too tired and hungry to argue about setting the table or complain about the meal. After dinner, an hour of television was enough to set sleepy heads nodding, and it was soon off to bed.

Today, however, it's not safe to turn children loose for an hour on their own, much less an entire day, so youngsters have fewer opportunities to work off excess energy. Economic conditions that have caused many mothers to enter the workforce have also contributed to the problems: a working mother's schedule doesn't leave time to dress and organize her distractible ADHD child for school each day, to pick up after him, take him back to school to retrieve forgotten books, and so on. When a family's schedule is planned down to the last minute, an ADHD youngster's problems can throw everything awry. Soon patience is exhausted, parents turn to professionals, and a diagnosis of ADHD is made in a youngster who might never have come to professional attention in the past.

Consider, too, the changes in school systems across the country. In years past, parents fought having their child labeled as a special-needs child, fearing that he would be stigmatized by such a label. Today, however, a child must have a label in order to receive resource services and classroom accommodations. Thus, parents are now more likely to seek a diagnostic evaluation if it means the child will get the help he needs in school.

In summary, many factors may explain the increase in the number of individuals diagnosed with ADHD. When all of these factors are taken into consideration, it would not appear that we are overdiagnosing ADHD. Instead, increased awareness has led to an appropriate increase in referrals and diagnoses. It's likely, as Dr. Swanson observed, that individuals with ADHD have been there all along but, until recently, their problems haven't been identified or treated.

CHAPTER 2

IS IT ONLY ADHD?

Subtypes and Related Learning, Emotional, and Behavioral Problems

Overview: Then and Now

Then: A decade ago, children with a wide array of problems were lumped together under the catchall diagnostic label "attention-deficit/hyperactivity disorder." It was—and is—confusing to parents that the same diagnostic label we apply to a boisterous, aggressive "whirling dervish" can also be applied to a shy, quiet daydreamer who appears to move through life in slow motion.

A decade ago, too, mental health professionals usually tried to find a single diagnosis to describe all the symptoms and difficulties that beset the child in front of them. This approach often led to more confusion than clarification because many children just do not fit neatly into a single diagnostic pigeonhole.

Now: We now know that there are very important differences between ADHD youngsters who are bouncy, active, and impulsive and those whose problems consist primarily of inattentiveness.

And, in what has been one of the most important advances in ADHD within the past decade, we have learned that individuals with ADHD are also likely to have other conditions and problems as well, a situation called "comorbidity." Comorbidity is important because it explains much of the confusion regarding diagnosis, prognosis, and treatment, as we will discuss.

Subtypes of ADHD

As we saw in Chapter 1, ADHD wears many faces—so many and so varied, in fact, that we cannot gain meaningful knowledge about ADHD by lumping individuals with such diverse problems into one big hodgepodge. Instead, we must divide ADHD individuals into smaller subgroups whose members have important features in common. But how should we define these subgroups?

One obvious distinction is that between youngsters who have attentional problems only (in DSM-IV terms, "ADHD, Predominantly Inattentive Type") and those whose attentional problems are accompanied by hyperactivity and impulsivity ("ADHD, Predominantly Hyperactive-Impulsive Type" and "ADHD, Combined Type"). Parents and teachers certainly have no difficulty telling the two groups apart: as one parent summarized succinctly, "Some are space cadets and some swing from the chandelier." Researchers, too, have found very important differences between the two groups, as discussed below.[13,14,15]

■ **Attention-Deficit/Hyperactivity Disorder, Predominantly Hyperactive-Impulsive Type and ADHD, Combined Type.** Formerly called attention deficit disorder *with* hyperactivity (ADD/H), these youngsters spring to mind when one hears the term hyperactive child. As a group, they are excessively active and impulsive. Many are also aggressive and their problems are usually apparent in a variety of settings. Their social relationships are often poor and they may be actively rejected and scapegoated by peers. Because adults find their behavior so annoying, these youngsters are often referred for professional help at an early age.

Even when they are referred early, however, some of these children do poorly because they tend to have coexisting oppositional defiant disorder and conduct disorder, both of which are difficult to treat (see below). If the child comes from a family in which there are multiple problems, such as parents or adult siblings with ADHD and/or substance abuse, treatment is even less likely to be successful.

Youngsters in this group may also have learning disabilities and many receive special education services in school. When they are placed in special classes, however, placement is most commonly in classrooms for behaviorally or emotionally disturbed students rather than in classes for learning-disabled children.

■ **Attention-Deficit/Hyperactivity Disorder, Predominantly Inattentive Type.** These children, formerly called attention deficit disorder *without* hyperactivity (ADD/WO), are at the opposite extreme from their hyperactive-impulsive counterparts in terms of activity. In fact, they tend to be somewhat sluggish and underactive in general tempo, and parents and teachers describe them as absentminded daydreamers and space cadets. Because they are often somewhat shy and socially withdrawn, they may have few friends. Many are rather clumsy, so they can't compensate for other deficits through sports.

These youngsters have problems with memory and with the speed with which they process information. They may be more prone to learning disabilities than their hyperactive counterparts and, when they receive special services in the school setting, it is likely to be in a classroom for learning-disabled students.

Anxiety disorders are common among children in this group, as well as in their family members. Some ADHD children with coexisting anxiety disorders respond well to treatment with stimulant medication, but others—perhaps the majority—have a poor response to stimulant medication when it is used alone (see Chapter 5).

Of course, not all ADHD children fall neatly into one of these two groups, but the distinction seems to be a useful one overall. In fact, many experts in the field of ADHD—Dr. Russell Barkley at the University of Massachusetts, Dr. Ben Lahey at the University of Georgia, and Dr. Caryn Carlson at the University of Texas among them—believe that ADD/H and ADD/WO are entirely separate disorders rather than subtypes of the same disorder. Evidence also suggests that the two disorders reflect problems in different areas of the brain and that different neurochemicals are involved as well.

I, too, believe that ADD/H and ADD/WO should be considered different disorders, especially after years of struggling to explain to parents of inattentive type youngsters that they should ignore the word "hyperactivity" in their child's diagnosis. I also think that this distinction will advance our knowledge about the causes of, and treatments for, both conditions.

Other distinctions also appear promising in terms of helping us understand and treat children with ADHD. We know, for example, that aggressive behavior in ADHD children is often associated with a worse outcome in life than we see in nonaggressive ADHD children. We also know that ADHD children who have a family history of ADHD are more likely to perform poorly on neuropsychological tests than those who do not have such a family history, suggesting that there are important differences between ADHD children with and without close relatives who have ADHD.[16]

Perhaps the single most important distinction that can be made among youngsters with ADHD at this time is the distinction between those with and without coexisting learning and psychiatric problems, as discussed in the following sections.

Comorbidity: Compounding the Confusion

We know that ADHD is one of the most common childhood psychiatric disorders, accounting for half or more of all referrals to child mental health services. Even today, however, the diagnosis of ADHD is not always clear-cut. The existence of comorbid conditions is still a major source of diagnostic confusion—and subsequent treatment failure—among children and adults with ADHD.

In the past, if a hyperactive, impulsive child also seemed depressed and anxious and had difficulty with his schoolwork, there might be lengthy debates among the professionals involved in the child's care. Depending upon each professional's area of expertise, very different explanations might be advanced to explain the child's problems.

DR. A: "He's hyperactive, all right. Look at what he did to my office! If that isn't ADHD, I don't know what is. *I think* it's ADHD."

DR. B: "No, I don't agree. *I think* he's just so anxious that he falls apart in new situations and that makes him wild."

DR. C: "Well, I can see that he's pretty wild. But I think that comes from the fact that he has to struggle so hard in school every day that he's running on overload. *I think* we're looking at the spillover from learning disabilities."

We now know that a very high percentage of ADHD children also have coexisting, or "comorbid," problems. This discovery marks a huge step forward in our knowledge. Since comorbid conditions can make a big difference in severity of symptoms and in how a child responds to particular medications, we can begin to understand why some ADHD children respond well to stimulant medication while others do not and why some ADHD children have a much bleaker prognosis than others. Unfortunately, new findings about high rates of comorbidity also mean that we must rethink much of what we believed we knew about ADHD. Just a decade ago, for example, most professionals believed that oppositional, defiant patterns of behavior were a component of ADHD. As I stated in *Your Hyperactive Child:** "Negativism, disobedience and a general attitude of 'I-don't-wanna-and-I'm-not-gonna!' are common features of (ADHD)." Today, however, we recognize this pattern as oppositional defiant disorder, a disorder that is entirely separate from ADHD, although the two often coexist.

Finally, new findings concerning comorbidity have important implications for diagnosis. Professionals who evaluate ADHD children should always be on the alert for other conditions that commonly coexist with ADHD, as we discuss in the following sections.

Comorbid Psychiatric Conditions

Researchers tell us that of ADHD children who are referred to mental health clinics, as many as two-thirds have at least one other psychiatric condition.[17] What are the specific psychiatric conditions most commonly associated with ADHD?

---

* New York: Doubleday, 1988.

Oppositional Defiant Disorder

Children with oppositional defiant disorder (ODD) are difficult children indeed. These are defiant, in-your-face, you-go-to-hell youngsters. As Dr. Bruce Pfeffer, a wise and experienced developmental pediatrician, so graphically summed up, ODD children seem to approach the world with their middle finger permanently extended!

Quarrelsome and spiteful, these youngsters often go out of their way to aggravate and annoy others without any provocation. Many express particular resentment—even outright hatred—toward siblings and constantly complain that their siblings are given preferential treatment. They may blame them for their own unhappiness: more than one ODD youngster has told me with obvious sincerity, "My life would be fine if it weren't for my brother" or "Everything would be great if I didn't have a sister."

These youngsters blame others, in addition to siblings, for their problems and lack insight into how they engineer their own difficulties. Like the ADHD child, they are argumentative, but, unlike the ADHD child, who seems to enjoy arguing simply as a sort of verbal Ping-Pong, ODD youngsters argue viciously, with anger and venom. Their tantrums, too, are different: while the ADHD child may fall apart and scream in frustration, the storm usually subsides quickly. ODD children escalate quickly into full-blown rage episodes, during which they may be physically assaultive, and brood and sulk for hours afterward.

Oppositional defiant disorder often emerges quite early in life. In fact, virtually all of the ODD children I've encountered started out as very difficult infants, became tyrannical toddlers, and went downhill from there. Research findings support my observations.

The youngest of three children, Carla was such a fretful, querulous infant that her parents, experienced as they were, felt overwhelmed by the demands of caring for her.

"She wasn't anything like the other two," her mother explained. "They had the normal baby stuff—fussy when they teethed or when they had a cold. But she was just an unhappy camper from the start, always had a scowl on her face. And it didn't get better as she got older:

it just got worse because she was bigger and could throw bigger tantrums. I hated to put my other two in preschool because I really enjoyed spending time with them. With Carla, I couldn't wait!"

One of the most baffling things about youngsters with ODD is the dramatic difference often observed between their public and private faces. In our book *Lonely, Sad and Angry: A Parent's Guide to Depression in Children and Adolescents*,★ Sam Goldstein and I commented:

> We have come away from more than one school conference about such children with the distinct impression that two entirely different children were discussed at the meeting: the well-behaved—even timid and submissive—child described by the teacher and the raging hell-terror we and the parents knew the child could often be at home.

What accounts for the difference in behavior at home and in school? Dr. Michel Maziade,[18] a psychiatrist in Quebec, believes that ODD children have a temperament characterized by predominantly negative mood, intense emotional reactions, and a tendency to withdraw in new situations. In school, where the ODD child must deal with new people and new situations, he quietly withdraws into his shell. In the familiar home setting, however, his high intensity and negative mood predispose him to angry, defiant, oppositional behavior.

I have long suspected that oppositional defiant disorder may be a variant of a mood disorder, since these children appear so angry and unhappy and since so many of them have a family history of mood disorders. Therefore, I was gratified to learn that other mental health professionals have noted this connection too: in a recent study of twenty-eight children diagnosed with ODD, low-grade depressive illness (dysthymia) was common.[19] It is of particular importance to note that in only one case was the child diagnosed with both ADHD and dysthymia at the time of the initial evaluation: in the remaining cases, the mood disorder had been overlooked at intake.

If ODD is not successfully treated during childhood, difficult behavior sometimes spills over into the school setting by the time the child enters

★ New York: Doubleday, 1995.

middle school. From there, it may be a downhill slide into the pattern of behavior seen in conduct disorder, described below.

Conduct Disorder

Conduct-disordered teenagers break rules and engage in antisocial behaviors that include lying, stealing, fighting, truancy, and running away from home. This profile calls to mind the kind of teenagers we used to call "juvenile delinquents," and "hoodlums"—the sort of kids your parents wouldn't let you date. Some conduct-disordered youngsters are bullies who intimidate and attack others. Some are deliberately cruel to animals and to other people and show little remorse for the harm they inflict. Conduct-disordered teens may also drink, smoke, use drugs, and engage in sexual activities at an early age and often in a promiscuous way.

"He's been nothing but trouble from as far back as I can remember. And, now that he's bigger, the troubles are bigger too." Ronald's mother sat in the doctor's office, nervously twisting a handkerchief as she talked.

"Even when he was little, he just couldn't seem to get along with the other kids and listen to the teacher. When he was in middle school, I got so many calls from the principal that I finally had him moved to another school. But it didn't work: he wasn't there a month before he got thrown out for smoking in the bathroom."

Pausing for a moment to collect her thoughts, she went on. "High school's been even worse. He's skipped a lot and he's hanging out with a nasty crowd. He stays out late—sometimes he doesn't come home at all. A week ago he came home drunk and I'm pretty sure he's into drugs." The tears glistening in her eyes ran down her cheeks. "But the thing that really scares me is that I think he's gotten involved with something illegal, something really bad. When I went to wash his clothes the other day, I found a big wad of money. He doesn't have any way to come by that money legally. What's he gotten himself into? What's going to happen to him?"

In its more serious forms, conduct disorder is very difficult to treat and some teenagers with conduct disorder go on to engage in antisocial behavior and criminal activities as adults. Parents, then, have every right to be worried if their ADHD youngster starts to show symptoms of conduct disorder, especially if the symptoms appear before age ten.

But before we conclude that all ADHD teens who violate the rules are on a fast track to the penitentiary, let's take a closer look. As Dr. Keith McBurnett[20] reminds us, many otherwise "good" teenagers dabble in milder forms of delinquent behaviors such as smoking, drinking underage, cutting classes, and staying out past curfew. Although they could be diagnosed with conduct disorder according to DSM-IV criteria, these youngsters are obviously very different from the more predatory youths who bully and attack others, set fires and vandalize property, and engage in other seriously antisocial acts. Teenagers in the former group tend to put aside their unacceptable behavior and join mainstream society, while many in the latter group go on to chronically antisocial and criminal lifestyles.

The ADHD child who is most likely to develop severe and persistent conduct disorder is one who has comorbid ODD and whose symptoms of conduct disorder appear in childhood. The risk is greater if he also has a mood disorder and/or learning disabilities (both of which commonly accompany conduct disorder), and greater still if his home life is unstable and chaotic and if members of his extended family have problems with substance abuse and antisocial behavior.

According to Dr. McBurnett, early warning signs that should alert you to trouble ahead include:

■ Angry, defiant behavior, blatant disregard for rules, and a taste for taking risks;
■ Physical fighting; rejection by "law-abiding" peers;
■ Persistent lying, cheating, and stealing;
■ Fascination with delinquent behavior, such as displaying symbols of gangs, acquiring forbidden objects like drug paraphernalia or pornography, and telling tales about real or imaginary antisocial feats.

If your child fits this pattern, run—don't walk—to a mental health professional who has expertise in working with children like yours. When conduct-disordered behavior is longstanding, it's particularly hard to change, so the earlier treatment starts, the better.

Mood Disorders

With all the difficulties ADHD children encounter with parents, teachers, and peers, it's not surprising that many of these youngsters become demoralized. What has come as a surprise to many professionals in the field, however, is the extent to which ADHD children and teenagers suffer from full-blown clinical depression.

Depression. Depression is *not* just a state of mind. It's an illness that affects every aspect of a person's life. People who suffer from depression don't just feel down or blue: depressed children, especially, are likely to be irritable, whiny, and prone to getting mired in bad moods. And it's not only the mind that is affected by depression, the body suffers too. Depressed children complain of aches and pains for which no medical cause can be found. They are also vulnerable to every bug that comes along, so they are often laid up with colds, strep infections, or the flu.

Depressed youngsters often have sleep problems such as difficulty falling asleep or repeated awakenings throughout the night. In either case, the youngster loses sleep time, so it isn't unusual to find that depressed children and adolescents complain of fatigue and low energy.

Like depressed adults, depressed children have a pessimistic outlook on life, always expecting the worst instead of the best. Nothing is much fun and few things arouse their interest because everything seems to require too much effort. They may withdraw from friends and social activities and go into a self-imposed "social hibernation." Sometimes life itself doesn't seem worth the effort and thoughts of death or dying present themselves as an alternative to the suffering they endure daily. In severe cases, a depressed person may attempt to take his own life.

From her self-description, no one would guess that nine-year-old Abigail was a pretty, bright youngster who did well in school and was liked by her classmates. "I'm not too smart," she explained. "And I'm not very pretty either. I know my parents are disappointed in me, even though they try to hide it. They're always trying to get me to call some friends or join a club or take some lessons."

"But," she sighed, "it really isn't any use: I wouldn't be good at anything. Anyway, most times I just don't feel like doing anything except maybe watch TV. Sometimes I'm so tired I don't even want to do that. And—I know this sounds awful—sometimes it seems like I don't even want to live anymore."

Depression, like other psychiatric disorders, tends to coexist with other psychiatric problems, and when it does, symptoms are generally more severe. Treatment, too, is more difficult than when depression exists without comorbid disorders.

Dysthymic Disorder. Children with dysthymic disorder resemble Eeyore, the character in the Winnie-the-Pooh stories who constantly brooded about feeling unloved and was generally irritable, gloomy, and low in self esteem. Unlike depression, dysthymic disorder is not characterized by loss of interest and pleasure or by social withdrawal or changes in sleep and appetite.

While less incapacitating than depression and therefore less obvious to the observer, dysthymic disorder is still a serious condition because it is often the forerunner of a full-blown depressive episode. Age of onset can be very early in life—so early that the symptoms seem to be a part of the individual's personality. Dysthymic disorder sometimes develops along with other chronic conditions, such as ADHD. In adolescents, it is closely associated with conduct disorder.

Bipolar Disorder. People with bipolar disorder (formerly called manic-depressive illness) alternate between periods of depression and manic periods in which mood and energy are excessively elevated. In manic periods, they may behave impulsively, taking serious risks without thought of consequences: they might, for example, go on spending sprees, invest in far-fetched business ventures, or suddenly declare mad, passionate love for the next-door neighbor. Some manic adults become so grandiose in their thinking that they act as if they were experts on subjects about which they know nothing or actually believe themselves to be some historical or religious figure, such as Mother Teresa or Jesus Christ.

In young people, mania and depression usually do not occur in clear and separate cycles. Instead, bipolar youngsters tend to have a mixture of chronic symptoms, of which irritability and rapid mood changes are the most prominent.

Until recently, bipolar disorder was believed to be quite rare in children. We now know, however, that at least one of every four children who suffers from depression will eventually develop bipolar disorder.[21] Those at greatest risk are youngsters with a history of severe hyperactivity, serious temper outbursts, and unstable mood, along with a family history of bipolar disorder and alcoholism.[22]

Anxiety Disorders

In a huge nationwide study, anxiety disorder emerged as the most common of the psychiatric disorders in the adult population. Of more than 17,000 adults surveyed, almost fifteen percent suffered from an anxiety disorder, and fully half of these individuals reported that their symptoms began before they were fifteen years old.[23] With the exception of ADHD, no other psychiatric disorder seen in adults has such an early age of onset. In fact, symptoms of some anxiety disorders can exist from the earliest months of life, as is sometimes the case with separation anxiety disorder.

Separation Anxiety Disorder. Some children with separation anxiety disorder never seem to outgrow the fear of being separated from parents that is normal in toddlers. When these children are separated from familiar people and surroundings, they protest with tears, tantrums, and wails of anguish. So fearful are they of separation that they may shadow a parent into the bathroom and insist on sharing the parental bed. Not surprisingly, school refusal, or "school phobia," is a common problem among youngsters with significant separation anxiety disorder. They often have other phobias as well, particularly phobias of injections and the sight of blood, and there is often much overlap with phobic disorder.

Phobic Disorder. Children with phobic disorder suffer from one or more intense irrational fears, known as phobias. Some phobias are common in the general population and generally cause little real distress: many people fear harmless snakes but their phobia doesn't interfere with their lives. Other phobias, however, can cause great distress, as in the case of a child who becomes hysterical at the sight of a bee or the threat of an injection. In some cases, phobias are so severe that exposure to the feared object or situation results in a *panic attack,* an episode of overwhelming anxiety accompanied by physical symptoms such as shortness of breath, rapid heartbeat, and feelings of being choked or smothered.

Generalized Anxiety Disorder. Because they are less spectacular, the symptoms of generalized anxiety disorder are not as obvious as those of separation anxiety disorder or phobic disorder, but they are no less troublesome to the child who suffers from them. Children with generalized anxiety disorder are tense, anxious perfectionists who stew and fret about almost everything imaginable. They are particularly likely to worry about whether their own performance will measure up, even in situations in which no one gives a hoot about "performance," so it's seldom that they can let down their hair and just have a good time.

> Eleven-year-old Michael, a poised and articulate youngster with an engaging manner, was quite open in describing his difficulties to the child psychologist. "I've been getting these weird feelings lately. They come over me a couple of times a day—anyway, at least once a day—and I feel really scared and alone and like something awful is going to happen, but I don't know what. And I worry a lot. In fact, I worry about just about everything you could think of. 'Will I pass my math test?' 'What if Mrs. Brenner calls on me in science and I don't know the answer?' 'What if my mom and dad were killed in an accident?' My brain just goes all the time and I can't stop it. I can't even stop it when I try to go to sleep."

Obsessive-Compulsive Disorder. Children with obsessive-compulsive disorder (OCD) are troubled by obsessions—persistent, unwanted thoughts or impulses that seem beyond their ability to control. Common obsessions include fear of contamination (contracting a fatal disease by touching a doorknob, for example); impulses to do something awful, like kick a puppy or scream obscenities in church; and doubts about things like having left a stove on or a door unlocked. As a result of obsessions, a person with OCD may feel compelled to perform certain acts (compulsions) such as repeatedly checking a door to be sure it is locked or scrubbing his hands after touching any object which might be "contaminated."

OCD is less common than the other anxiety disorders and, when it occurs, it is often associated with a mood disorder or another anxiety disorder. Obsessive-compulsive behavior is also a feature of Tourette's syndrome (see below).

Anxiety disorders often coexist with each other and with mood disorders. When they accompany a mood disorder, the mood disorder is more severe and more difficult to treat.[24] Finally, like ADHD, anxiety disorders tend to be chronic, although symptoms of separation anxiety disorder may wax and wane over time and children with this disorder may go into long periods of remission.

Community surveys indicate that about one-third of children with ADHD have comorbid anxiety disorders, a figure that is quite high indeed.[25] A comorbid anxiety disorder greatly complicates treatment in ADHD children because many of these youngsters have a rather poor response to stimulant medication (see Chapter 5).

Tic Disorders

Tics are sudden involuntary motor movements such as eye-blinking, neck-jerking, and facial grimaces, or sudden involuntary sounds such as throat-clearing, sniffing, and barking noises. Some tics are transient in nature; others persist over time. In Tourette's syndrome there are multiple and persistent motor and vocal tics which, when the condition is severe, interfere with the individual's ability to function in society. Children with tic disorder usually have other problems as well and, for many, these problems are generally more troublesome than their tics. More than fifty percent have ADHD and many also have obsessive-compulsive disorder, depression, and problems with aggression. The more severe the tics, the more severe and complex the associated problems tend to be.[26]

A small percentage of ADHD children have episodic motor or vocal tics, generally mild in nature. A smaller percentage suffer from full-blown Tourette's syndrome. Since symptoms of ADHD often emerge much earlier in life than symptoms of Tourette's syndrome, some youngsters with Tourette's syndrome may be erroneously diagnosed as having only ADHD.

Learning Disabilities

Even ADHD youngsters who are intellectually gifted often perform poorly in school. Sometimes a learning problem is glaringly obvious, as when a bright, motivated child cannot master basic reading skills, despite his best efforts. In other cases, the child's report card is a crazy-quilt of grades ranging from A's to F's for no apparent reason.

As Priscilla Vail points out,[27] the learning and performance profiles of these children are so jagged and irregular that they resemble a cross-section of the Alps. One child, for example, may have an excellent vocabulary and command of the language, yet fail miserably when asked to put his thoughts on paper. Another might have strong skills in reading and written language but fall apart in math. Others have excellent conceptual abilities but lack skills in spelling or language mechanics so others can't make sense of their written work. Still others, bright enough to compensate for learning difficulties, falter when they encounter the demands of middle school. It is these "conundrum kids" who confound parents and educators and whose problems are often attributed to laziness, stubbornness, and lack of motivation.

Learning Difficulties and Disabilities in ADHD

There is no question that ADHD children often have difficulty with academic performance. In fact, the statistics are rather grim: up to eighty percent of ADHD children seen in clinical settings have academic achievement problems and many repeat at least one grade or are placed in special education settings.[28]

How many ADHD youngsters have learning disabilities? The answer depends on how one defines a learning disability. The term "learning disabled" refers to children who fail to learn at an expected rate despite an apparently normal capacity for learning. Thus, in order for a child to be diagnosed as learning disabled, there must be a significant discrepancy between the child's scores on intelligence tests (his "capacity" for learning) and his scores on academic achievement tests (his actual level of academic performance) in one or more of six areas:

- Oral expression
- Listening comprehension
- Written expression
- Basic reading skills
- Mathematics calculation
- Mathematical reasoning

If we consider a twenty-point discrepancy between IQ scores and achievement scores to indicate a "significant discrepancy," as is currently the general practice, we find that fewer than ten percent of children in the U.S. can be diagnosed as learning disabled. Among ADHD children, the figure jumps to about twenty to twenty-five percent or higher.[29]*

Why is there so much overlap between ADHD and learning disabilities? In the past, some thought that the learning problems of many ADHD children were caused by their inattentiveness. Others argued the reverse; that learning difficulties actually caused inattentiveness and restlessness.

There is probably a grain of truth in both of these arguments: Certainly the inattentiveness and sloppy, disorganized work habits of untreated ADHD children often contribute to poor academic achievement. Conversely, in order to avoid struggling with work beyond his abilities, the learning-disabled youngster might gaze out the window, leave his seat, and chat with other students in class.

We now know, however, that while the two conditions commonly coexist, they are separate disorders. Like ADHD, learning disabilities tend to run in families and, like ADHD, learning disabilities are thought to result from differences in brain anatomy and chemistry (see Chapter 4). The most common learning disabilities—those which involve reading—appear to stem from problems in the left hemisphere of the brain, the part of the brain that is specialized for language. Less common are the nonver-

---

* It's important to note that these figures do *not* take into account children who have a less-than-twenty-point discrepancy between IQ and achievement test scores but who still have significant difficulty with learning problems. Although these children are legion, because they do not meet the criteria to be labeled learning disabled, many fail to receive the services they need to help them learn and achieve. These are truly children who "fall between the cracks."

bal learning disabilities, which appear to stem from problems in the right hemisphere, the part of the brain that is specialized for visual/spatial information.

■ **Language-Based Learning Disabilities.** Reading disorders, sometimes referred to as "dyslexia," do not stem from problems with visual perception, as some have assumed. Instead, dyslexic individuals most commonly have problems with language processing. In particular, they have trouble learning the code that links the forty or so basic sounds of our language (phonemes) and the twenty-six letters of our alphabet.

Individuals who can't easily master this code have difficulty decoding written words quickly and automatically when reading. The effort involved in decoding the words distracts them from the meaning of what they read so they must read the same sentence or paragraph over and over to derive meaning.

People with these "phonological processing" problems also have problems putting words into written form (encoding) as well. They struggle with spelling and with written work in general.

Children with language-based learning disabilities often have difficulty memorizing things in sequence, such as the days of the week. They also have particular problems memorizing math facts and remembering the sequence of steps involved in math computation.

■ **Nonverbal Learning Disabilities.** Children with nonverbal learning disabilities have difficulty organizing visual information and coordinating visual information with motor activity. They have a poor grasp of spatial relationships—where one object is relative to another—so they can't gauge direction and distance. Directional differences between letters (b and d; m and w) confuse them, as do sequencing differences (was vs. saw) so they may read "I saw a dog" as "I was a god."

Children with nonverbal learning disabilities have difficulty developing a sight vocabulary and so must sound out each word instead of recognizing common words at a glance. Thus, reading is a time-consuming process during which the reader can lose the meaning of what he is decoding, a word at a time.

Children with poor visual memory have problems with spelling because they can't tell when a word doesn't look right. They have problems with writing, too, especially if they have poor visual-motor coordination.

The struggles with the mechanical skills of writing may be so great that the child resists writing more than the minimum needed to get by.

Outside of the classroom, people with nonverbal learning disabilities have problems reading maps and become lost in all but the most familiar surroundings. A child who can't judge the distance to home plate or gauge the speed of the ball coming at him won't have much success on the athletic field. A person who can't detect important nonverbal cues in social interaction is likely to have problems with social skills and interpersonal relationships.

Developmental Speech and Language Disorders

Over a decade ago, it was discovered that ADHD children have an unusually high rate of speech and language disorders, many of which go undetected and, therefore, untreated. Since then, researchers have confirmed that as many as half or more of all children referred to mental health settings for treatment of ADHD have such problems.[30]

Children with ADHD very commonly have problems with speech articulation—mispronouncing certain letters and combinations of letters. Many have expressive language difficulties such as word-finding problems (thinking of the word or phrase to express a thought) as well as problems formulating fluent and grammatically correct sentences and putting sentences together into a coherent narrative. Some also have problems with receptive language; that is, they can't understand, organize, or remember what they hear. These children commonly have problems with phonological processing (ability to distinguish between speech sounds), a problem that in turn interferes with their ability to grasp basic-sound symbol relationships needed for reading.

Children who have receptive language problems may be diagnosed by speech pathologists with "central auditory processing disabilities." Since children with CAPD are often described as inattentive and distractible, it is not surprising to find that there is a great deal of overlap between ADHD and CAPD and that it is sometimes quite difficult to distinguish between the two conditions.[31]

Although ADHD toddlers are more likely than others to be delayed in talking, when they begin to talk, it's as if they were trying to make up for lost time, so chatty and talkative are they. But because they have word-finding difficulties as well as problems organizing their thoughts, they may find it difficult to respond quickly to direct questions. This explains why a child who talks your ear off for an hour about his favorite video game suddenly clams up and becomes the Great Stone Face when you ask him a simple question like "What did you do in school today?"

In conversation, the ADHD child finds it hard to stay on a single topic and, because he is inattentive, he often does not hear or acknowledge what the other person says. Since it is difficult for him to wait for his turn, he may butt in before the other person has finished, sometimes with something wildly off topic. These are not the hallmarks of a brilliant conversationalist!

Problems in getting their thoughts together to put them into words are often painfully obvious in ADHD children.[32] When the ADHD child attempts to recount an experience, his tale may be so disorganized that the listener is quickly lost in a verbal maze.

> "That movie was so cool! This guy—um, he was an alien—came to earth because they were all going to die without this stuff they needed for—uh—whatever. And his girlfriend got killed by the other guys—the Zogars. Only she wasn't really killed but they—um, see—they thought she was. But, then—oh, and he had this really neat thing like a mirror except not really but when he used it, it made everybody invisible except she could see him but they—no, wait: he could see her but they had to have this thing that the other guys had to see them. And they needed this stuff from earth but—no—I forgot: before that, they . . ."

When this young movie critic is asked to summarize the story his class has just read, how do you think he will fare?

Outside the classroom, too, the ability to tell a story, give directions, or recount an experience are important in daily social interaction. The child who rambles on in such a disjointed fashion will quickly lose the attention and interest of his listeners.

What Causes the Problem?

From the discussion above, you can see that some of the speech/language problems of ADHD children may be due to difficulties with planning, organization, inattentiveness, and impulsivity. Other problems, however, probably reflect specific dysfunctions in the left hemisphere of the brain, the part of the brain that is specialized for language. It may be, too, that some ADHD youngsters develop receptive and expressive language disorders as a result of chronic ear infections that interfere with early opportunities to learn speech and language (see below).

Whatever the cause, suspected developmental language problems in an ADHD child should be evaluated by a competent speech pathologist. With the exception of articulation problems (difficulty pronouncing certain speech sounds), speech and language problems don't go away with maturation, so the child with a language disorder doesn't catch up as he grows up.[33] Since developmental speech and language problems are often associated with learning disabilities as well as with school refusal,[34] they are not something to be taken lightly.

Medical Problems and Physical Anomalies

As noted in Chapter 1, young ADHD children are particularly prone to upper respiratory infections and ear infections. In fact, ADHD children are twice as likely as others to have a history of chronic middle ear infections with fluid behind the eardrum, a condition that often requires the surgical insertion of tubes to allow the fluid to drain.[35] These recurrent infections suggest problems with the immune system in ADHD children and, in fact, researchers report that ADHD children have lower levels of a particular blood protein known as C4B, which defends the body from viral and bacterial infections.[36] Might this deficiency actually be a cause of ADHD in some ADHD children, or is it merely a "marker" for ADHD? The answer at this time is not known, but we can certainly expect clarification in the very near future.

Although research findings are mixed, ADHD children also seem prone to allergies. This observation has led some to conclude that ADHD can be treated by treating suspected allergies to certain foods and chemicals by means of controlled diets such as the Feingold Diet and other allergy treatment programs. In general, this approach to treating ADHD has proved quite disappointing.

On the other hand, ADHD children do not have higher rates of asthma than children in the general population, as was previously thought to be the case, nor do standard treatments for asthma result in ADHD-like symptoms.[37] In fact, asthma is more closely linked with anxiety disorders, so an asthmatic child suspected of having ADHD should also be examined closely for the presence of such disorders.

Several researchers have found that ADHD children often have minor abnormalities in motor, sensory, and integrative functions—abnormalities such as poor fine-motor coordination, clumsiness, poor balance, impaired hand-eye coordination, and irregular, jerky movements. These neurological "soft signs" reflect a primary disturbance in the central nervous system, so it is not surprising that they are common among ADHD children, as ADHD itself is due to CNS dysfunction or difference. However, these soft signs are of little help in making a diagnosis of ADHD, since they are also associated with learning disabilities and with a number of other psychiatric disorders.

ADHD children also have a high incidence of minor physical abnormalities such as widely spaced eyes, low-set and abnormally shaped ears, and abnormal palmar creases. These minor physical anomalies are observed not only in ADHD children but in their biological relatives as well, pointing to a genetic origin. In fact, the research of Dr. Curtis Deutsch at Harvard Medical School suggests that both the physical abnormalities and the attentional and behavioral problems seen in ADHD stem from the same genetically determined maldevelopment of the brain.[38]

While not medical problems in the strict sense, problems with sleep and elimination (wetting and soiling) are also common in ADHD children. Sleep problems usually involve difficulty falling asleep and may worsen when the child is treated with stimulant medication. Problems with wetting and soiling when other children have mastered control of these bodily functions pose just one more threat to self-esteem in children whose self-esteem is already at an ebb.

Social Problems

In play with their peers, children learn such critical life skills as cooperation, negotiation, and how to settle disputes—skills that they cannot learn or practice in their nonegalitarian relationships with adults. In playing with other children, opportunities arise to engage creativity in fantasy play and to learn how to "pick up" on the unstated rules for interacting with others.

When children are rejected or ignored by other children, they miss out on important learning experiences that prepare one for later life. They miss out, too, on much of the fun and enjoyment of childhood and suffer the pangs all humans feel when they are rejected and unwanted by others.

Poor peer relationships don't just cause emotional pain and suffering during childhood: they are red flags that signal a risk for serious difficulties in later life. We don't yet know whether early social problems actually cause later adjustment problems or whether they are only "markers" that indicate problems ahead. We do know that compared with their more accepted peers, children with social problems are more likely to drop out of school, engage in antisocial behavior, and have mental health problems as adults.[39]

As noted in preceding sections, ADHD children often have serious difficulties getting along with other children. Some, like the quiet, retiring youngsters with ADHD/inattentive type, are just ignored by their peers and left to go their lonely way undisturbed. Often, however—especially in the case of ADHD children who are impulsive and hyperactive—they are actively disliked, rejected, and picked on by peers.

What is there about ADHD children that causes them to have problems connecting with their peers? For some inattentive type ADHD children, their shyness and general "spaciness" are obstacles to forming friendships. Those who are hyperactive and impulsive may be so bossy, impulsive, intrusive, and aggressive that peers shy away or become aggressive in turn. Poor language skills undoubtedly play a role in the social isolation and rejection of some ADHD youngsters, while an inability to pick up on subtle social cues prevents many from being accepted by other children.

Whatever the source of the child's interpersonal difficulties, it is important to address the problem, since successful interaction with others is the basis for virtually all success and satisfaction in life. The problem of poor social skills is discussed at length in Chapter 7.

CHAPTER 3

DOES MY CHILD HAVE ADHD? DO I HAVE IT TOO?

Overview: Then and Now

Then: A decade ago, many professionals still based a diagnosis of ADHD on the child's behavior in the office. If the child didn't demolish the office, attack other children in the waiting room, or bite the nurse, the verdict was likely to be "not hyperactive."

Parents, too, were much less knowledgeable a decade ago than they are now. Many found it difficult to understand how a youngster who could remain glued to television for hours might have problems with attention and concentration. Others, confused by terminology, were puzzled at the idea that a shy, quiet daydreamer could have anything in common with "hyperactive" children.

There was also limited awareness of the extent of the problem in the adult population. In fact, some practitioners were still assuring parents that their children would outgrow their symptoms of ADHD in adolescence. A few pioneering scientists, like Dr. Paul Wender at the University of Utah, insisted that ADHD symptoms continued well into the adult years but, for the most part, adult ADHD was terra incognita, unknown territory.

Now: Parents and professionals know much more about ADHD now than they did ten years ago. Along with this knowledge has come an appreciation for the difficulties involved in diagnosing ADHD. Many pediatricians now refer these youngsters to mental health professionals with specific expertise in assessing ADHD. If pediatricians conduct their own evaluations, they usually schedule an extended appointment for the child and avail themselves of rating scales and other assessment devices that can help in the identification of ADHD.

Adults with ADHD, too, have been recognized as a population with special needs. Support groups have sprung up all over the country; an annual conference is held on adult ADHD; and several excellent books on the subject have been published.

A Comprehensive Evaluation: Don't Leave Home Without One

Since a treatment plan is only as good as the diagnosis on which it is based, it's crucial to obtain the best evaluation possible. Unfortunately, in the attempt to obtain a good evaluation, parents may go from one narrowly focused specialist to another. Too often, the result is a fat collection of documents that provides little in the way of real help to the child.

When Mrs. Henderson called to make an appointment for her son, Dr. Stewart started to explain his evaluation procedure but Mrs. Henderson cut him off. "We don't need an evaluation," she explained. "Stefan has already been diagnosed with ADHD. We just need some new ideas for treatment, because nothing we've tried seems to work."

An alarm sounded in the back of Dr. Stewart's mind. If Stefan had been correctly diagnosed, why hadn't any interventions been helpful? From experience, he knew that most ADHD children would respond at least moderately well to stimulant medication. And behavior management techniques—sometimes surprisingly simple ones—had helped many an ADHD child achieve success at home and in school. "What's going on here?" he wondered.

When the Hendersons arrived in his office with reports from the professionals who had evaluated Stefan, Dr. Stewart had his answer. Stefan had been tested, assessed, and examined by a host of competent professionals, but each had assessed Stefan only from the perspective of a single specialty. No one had assembled the pieces into a "big picture" so, like the blind men who each grabbed a different part of the elephant, the result was utter confusion instead of a carefully coordinated treatment plan.

Unfortunately, too, the result may be a child who is weary of being tested and parents who have drained their purses without having much to show for their efforts. The plight of these families underscores the wisdom of Dr. Michael Gordon's advice to parents in his book, *ADHD/ Hyperactivity: A Consumer's Guide*.* In big bold letters on the very first page, Dr. Gordon exhorts parents "SEEK THE BEST IN EVALUATION BEFORE YOU SEEK THE BEST IN TREATMENT." This is very good advice indeed.

Components of a Comprehensive Evaluation

When a parent says "My child has been diagnosed with ADHD," this can mean that the child has had anything from a brief office visit with his pediatrician to an exhaustive series of tests, including a physical exam, blood work and urinalysis, an EEG, neuropsychological testing, a speech-language evaluation, and psychiatric interview.

What do you really need in the way of an evaluation? Is a fifteen-minute interview with a pediatrician enough? Are EEGs useful? What about psychological testing? What about neuropsychological testing?

The best evaluation is not necessarily the most time-consuming or the most expensive. It does, however, involve more than a brief office visit and a cursory review of teacher rating scales. At a minimum, an evaluation should include a thorough review of the child's history and family history; detailed information about his past and current performance at home and in school; and a clinical interview with the child and the parents.

Let's take a closer look at each of these components.

* DeWitt, N.Y.: GSI Publications, 1991.

Taking a History: The Parent Interview

Many professionals—I am one of them—meet with the parents alone at the first visit to obtain background information about the child. This spares the child the humiliation of sitting there while three adults discuss his shortcomings and failures.* It also allows parents to speak freely about personal or family problems without the child present.

At this visit, the professional will gather information about your child's health and medical history, his motor and language development, his psychological history, and his educational experiences. You will be asked many questions about other members of the family too:

- If there are brothers and sisters, are they doing well socially and academically?
- Have any family members been diagnosed with ADHD, learning disabilities, depression, anxiety disorders, alcoholism, or other psychiatric problems? Even if a formal diagnosis has not been made, are there family members who have had difficulty in these areas?
- How do you and your spouse get along? Who is the disciplinarian in the family? Do parents agree on discipline and rules?

In Appendix A there is a developmental history questionnaire to help you organize information about your child and your family. In addition to such a questionnaire, the professional will probably ask you to complete other questionnaires and rating scales. Some will be difficult to complete, particularly if you yourself have ADHD. Steel yourself to do your best, because the quality of information you provide will directly affect the accuracy of the diagnosis.

You should also prepare a file containing your child's academic records. Include all report cards, results of standardized testing, and reports from other mental health professionals, tutors, speech pathologists, occupational therapists, and others who have evaluated or worked with your child in the past. This file should also include recent samples of the

---

* No wonder young people often refuse to attend follow-up sessions with mental health professionals if this has been their introduction to working with these professionals!

child's schoolwork. (If you do not have such a file, now is the time to start one!)

Don't leave original papers and reports with the professional. Instead, make legible copies of all material in the file. Add any notations you think might be helpful and arrange the material in chronological order before giving the file to the professional. The groundwork for the first appointment is tedious and time-consuming, but the effort you expend will reap dividends in terms of an accurate diagnosis for your child.

Observing Behavior in the Environment: Rating Scales

The professional will also want to know how your child functions in different settings. (In fact, as noted in Chapter 1, DSM-IV criteria *require* that symptoms be observed in more than one setting in order for a diagnosis of ADHD to be made.)

It would be prohibitively expensive to have a professional observe the child's behavior at home, in school, and in other settings. For this reason, professionals obtain information through rating scales completed by parents, teachers, baby-sitters, and others who can report on the child's typical behavior in different settings.

Rating scales provide a great deal of information in condensed form. They also permit comparison of your child's behavior with that of his age mates. By examining your child's score on a standardized rating scale, your doctor can say, for example, "In terms of attention span, he has a lower rating than ninety-five percent of children his age."

Some of the most widely used rating scales for parents are the Conners' Parent Rating Scale (Revised), the Child Behavior Checklist, the Home Situations Questionnaire, and the Attention Deficit Disorders Evaluation Scale. Rating scales for teachers include the Conners' Teacher Rating Scale (Revised), the ADD-H Comprehensive Teacher's Rating Scale (ACTeRS), and the School Situations Questionnaire. On these scales, the observer rates the child on a numerical scale on behaviors such as "Disturbs other children" and "Works well independently." Some scales yield a single summary score. Others, like the ACTeRS, yield separate scores for attention, hyperactivity, and social skills.

Although rating scales can yield useful information, they are subjective measures, that is, the rater must use his judgment to score particular behaviors. Thus, a doting grandmother might assign a score of zero, indicating "no problem," when asked to rate her grandson on the item "Disturbs others." On the other hand, a harried kindergarten teacher who has to deal with the child's restless and impulsive behavior in a class of twenty little five-year-olds might assign the same child a much higher score because she sees the problem as quite significant.

The problem is also complicated by the fact that the ADHD child's behavior can vary considerably across settings. In fact, in about one-fourth of clinic-referred ADHD children, we find considerable differences between teacher ratings and parent ratings. Sometimes, too, there are discrepancies between parents or between a teacher and a day-care provider. When this happens, we must try to understand why the child's behavior appears so different across circumstances and/or observers. My clinical experience suggests the following rough rules of thumb.

- Some discrepancies between parent ratings are to be expected, since mothers and fathers view their children from different perspectives and since children often behave better for Dad than for Mom. However, when the ratings are very different—when one parent rates the child a saint while the other sees him as a devil—I suspect a hidden agenda. In my experience, this pattern is most common in divorced or soon-to-be-divorced parents who can be counted on to enter into fierce custody battles. Each parent has a vested interest in his or her own point of view, so ratings will be skewed accordingly.

Through clenched teeth, Mrs. Hopkins described the legal battles she faced with her former husband. "He's furious that I finally got fed up enough to leave him and he plans to use Adam to get back at me. He knows as well as I do that Adam's always had problems. But it looks a lot better in court to say that Adam was a perfectly normal child until his selfish mother—meaning me—decided to destroy his happy home. There's no way he'll admit that Adam's always been a handful: that's not the case he plans to present to the judge."

- When teacher ratings indicate severe problems but parent ratings indicate only mild problems, the discrepancy might reflect a poor teacher-child relationship or it could signal a learning disability that causes the child to be particularly inattentive and disruptive in school.

The discrepancy could also reflect competent parents who don't consider their child's behavior problematic. Of course, behavior that is okay at home may be quite unacceptable in a classroom of twenty children.

With his curly hair and dimples, five-year-old Joey was the image of the all-American boy. Cute as she found him, however, the child psychologist grew increasingly uneasy as Joey disassembled the contents of her bookcases and used the empty shelves as a jungle gym while the psychologist talked with his mother. Finally, she spoke up. "What do you do when Joey does this at home? Doesn't it bother you?" she asked Joey's mother.

"Oh, no, not at all" was the reply. "Whenever he gets too wild, I just open the back door, whistle, and holler, 'You! Out! Now!' Then he goes out and runs around for a while until he's too tired to do much more than flop on the couch." She thought for a moment, then went on. "But I guess his teacher can't do that with him, can she?"

▪ What about situations in which parents describe severe problems but teachers report no difficulty? This may be a red flag for a diagnosis of oppositional defiant disorder.

Carla was a model of deportment in second grade, just as she had been in first grade. In fact, her second-grade teacher described her as "almost too good." At home, however, it was quite a different story. From the time Carla got off the bus in the afternoon to the time she went to bed, she seemed to be spoiling for a fight. If her mother asked how her day went, she received a snarl in response. But, if her mother said nothing when Carla entered the house, that was also grounds for complaint. Weekends were no better: No matter what the plans were, Carla complained and argued. As her father remarked, "She's the only kid I know who can pout about a trip to an amusement park or sulk all the way home from a birthday party."

Observing the Child: The Child Interview

Like adults, children deserve the privacy of an individual interview. Most actually appreciate an opportunity to talk about their difficulties with a concerned professional. While some youngsters are guarded and a few are outright hostile, the majority are relieved that someone is willing to listen and hear their side of the story. Many, in fact, spontaneously ask when they can come back again, and hover anxiously as their parents make a follow-up appointment.

How should you prepare your child for the interview? Most children are well aware of their difficulties. If a child is always in trouble for failing to complete his schoolwork, he knows that this is a problem. If he has peer problems, he knows that, too, although he may be too embarrassed to admit it. You've certainly talked about these problems with your child, so a general reference to his difficulties is usually sufficient, along with telling him that he will talk with someone who knows how to help children with problems like his.

The format of the interview varies from professional to professional, but it is standard practice to gather information about how the child functions in school.

- How do you get along with your teacher and your classmates?
- Is the work hard or easy?
- Is it hard for you to pay attention and keep your mind on your work?

Some children can recognize and describe their difficulties, but an experienced professional won't be surprised if the child denies or minimizes the problems reported by his parents and teachers, nor will he conclude that the child is lying. Even bright ADHD children may lack insight into their own behavior and how it appears to others, so their self-reports may be unreliable.

Family relationships will be explored too. And whether or not the parents have reported symptoms of anxiety or depression, a careful interviewer will inquire about these issues, since even the most concerned and caring parent may not be fully aware of the child's fears, anxieties, self-dislike, and sad moods.

In the interview, an astute clinician will be alert to various aspects of the child's behavior. Does the child separate easily from his parents in the waiting room, or does he cling anxiously to a parent? Is he friendly and chatty or quiet and reserved? Can he stay on a topic or does he tend to go into rambling discourses unrelated to the subject? Does he remain seated or dart about the office? How difficult is it to engage or redirect the child's attention? Are speech and language appropriate for the child's age? Is it difficult to understand him?

What if your child is uncooperative and difficult at this appointment? As embarrassing as this might be, it lets the professional see your child "in action," and that can be a valuable source of information. However, if the child is clearly out of control, it is better to remove him from the situation than to continue to put pressure on an already-stressed youngster.

Evaluating the Child: Diagnostic Tests

In this high-tech age, many parents are dismayed to learn that no laboratory tests can confirm a diagnosis of ADHD. In spite of exciting developments in brain imaging that have advanced our knowledge about ADHD, we still don't have a "litmus test" for ADHD.

Since conclusive medical tests are not yet available, can we use psychological tests to aid in making the diagnosis? The answer, as we shall see, is a carefully qualified yes.

For our purposes, we can roughly divide the psychological tests that might be used in diagnosing ADHD into four categories: tests of intelligence and academic achievement, neuropsychological tests, personality tests, and continuous performance tests.

Tests of Intelligence and Achievement. With children between the ages of six and sixteen, the most commonly used intelligence test is the Wechsler Intelligence Scale for Children, Third Edition, often referred to as the "WISC III." Currently, the most widely used tests of academic achievement are the Woodcock-Johnson Psychoeducational Battery, the Peabody Individual Achievement Test, and Wide Range Achievement Test (Revised).

Neither intelligence tests nor tests of academic achievement are particularly helpful in diagnosing ADHD, although behavioral observations made during testing can be enlightening. However, when school performance is a problem, as it so often is with ADHD youngsters, these tests can provide valuable information. For this reason, many professionals include intelligence and achievement testing as part of their diagnostic workup.

According to federal law, these tests must be provided by the public school system when a learning disability is suspected (see Chapter 9). Since insurance seldom covers these costly tests, many parents opt to have the testing done through the public school system. Some, however, are wary of professionals employed by the school system: "How do I know that I can trust them?" they ask. Since school psychologists are bound by a professional code of ethics, it would be virtually unthinkable to falsify test results. However, there may be considerable room for disagreement in how the test results are interpreted. If this appears to be the case, a second opinion can be obtained from a private psychologist concerning interpretation of test results, an approach which is much less expensive than having the tests themselves administered privately.

Neuropsychological Tests. These tests were originally designed to diagnose and assess brain damage and to serve as tools in research on brain-behavior relationships. They include tests of cognition, memory, attention, auditory and visual processing, and strategic planning.

Because ADHD involves dysfunction in the frontal lobes of the brain (see Chapter 4), some professionals use neuropsychological tests of frontal lobe functioning to help diagnose ADHD. On the face of it, this would appear to make good sense, but experts disagree as to the value of such tests. As Dr. Russell Barkley points out, these tests may show differences between groups of individuals with ADHD and those without, and yet be poor at classifying or diagnosing specific individuals.[40] Therefore, Dr. Barkley argues that they are not likely to be of value in diagnosing ADHD.

On the other hand, the group at Harvard University led by Doctors Joseph Biederman and Stephen Faraone[41] have found a pattern of neuro-psychological test results that seems to be consistent in ADHD children. These results are particularly pronounced in ADHD children with a family history of ADHD and they seem to be specific to ADHD; that is, they are not associated with any comorbid psychiatric conditions that might exist.

What should we conclude? At this time, neuropsychological testing can be helpful in pinpointing strengths and weaknesses for treatment planning—few would argue with this conclusion. However, in an age of tight budgets and limited insurance reimbursement, these expensive tests should not be routinely used in an evaluation for ADHD.

Personality Tests. Personality tests include self-report inventories and questionnaires, often in true-false or multiple choice format. While these measures are not helpful in diagnosing ADHD, they can provide information about how the child sees himself and his world. They can also help identify particular concerns and problems. When a mood disorder is suspected, for example, but the child has a hard time expressing his thoughts and feelings clearly, the Children's Depression Inventory offers the child a variety of options from which to select (e.g., "I am sad once in a while" vs. "I am sad many times" vs. "I am sad all the time"). Often, a youngster's response to a specific item will serve as a springboard for a discussion that yields further insights into the child's difficulties.

On the other hand, I do not find so-called "projective" personality tests to be helpful, either in making a diagnosis or in understanding the psychological functioning of an individual child. Projective tests such as the Rorschach Inkblot Technique or the Children's Thematic Apperception Test require the child to use his imagination to see shapes in the inkblots or make up stories about pictures. Some clinicians believe that the child's responses offer a window into his inner world of fears, needs, and fantasies. Others, like myself, prefer to use more direct means of obtaining information about the child, especially when diagnostic decisions are involved.

Continuous Performance Tests. Continuous performance tests (CPTs) can help pinpoint problems of attention, concentration, and impulsivity with children and adults in whom ADHD is suspected. Two such CPTs, the Conners' Continuous Performance Test and the Test of Variables of Attention (TOVA), are administered on a computer; a third, the Gordon Diagnostic System, presents the "targets" on the screen of a portable, self-contained unit.

All three CPTs require the child to watch closely as letters, numbers, or geometric figures are presented continuously, each target appearing briefly on the screen. On the TOVA and the Gordon, the child's task is to press a response button only when specific targets appear and to refrain from responding to all other targets. On the Conners', the reverse is true: the child is instructed to press a button in response to all nontargets and to refrain from responding when the identified target appears.

Experts disagree about whether these tests are helpful in diagnosing

ADHD. I have used one CPT for ten years and recently added a second one to my assessment battery. I find that these tests often enhance my understanding of how an individual approaches new tasks, how well he is able to stick with a boring task, how well he can control restlessness and impulsive responding over time, and so on. I also find that the results can be quite helpful in explaining a diagnosis of ADHD and in monitoring a child's response to medication (see Chapter 5).

Nevertheless, a word of caution is very much in order here! CPTs, like any other tool, are only as good as the person who uses them. The information they provide is only one small piece of the diagnostic puzzle, so they should *never* be used in isolation (as in "screening" for ADHD) and they should *never* be interpreted by anyone other than an experienced, well-trained professional.

Other Diagnostic Tests. Some parents ask if the tests employed in brain research studies of ADHD individuals are available to their children. These tests and the information about ADHD that they have provided are truly exciting. Unfortunately, however, their use remains limited to research settings at this time either because of the prohibitive expense involved or because, while they are useful tools for studying differences between groups of children, they are not yet helpful in diagnosing an individual child.

Medical laboratory tests such as blood work and urinalysis are of no help in diagnosing ADHD, nor are they needed before prescribing stimulant medication (although they are necessary if medications other than the stimulants are prescribed). Among children in whom ADHD is suspected, the results of a physical examination are usually completely normal. It is necessary, however, to rule out a physical cause such as lead poisoning or thyroid abnormalities, although these conditions are extremely rare and almost never explain the child's ADHD symptoms.

If the exam includes a neurological screening, the physician might observe the neurological soft signs and/or the minor physical anomalies described in Chapter 2. This is valuable information, but neither soft signs nor minor physical anomalies are diagnostic of ADHD, since they occur in other conditions as well.

Neither an evaluation by a neurologist nor an EEG (electroencephalogram) is necessary unless there is good reason to suspect a seizure disorder (epilepsy) or a progressive disease of the central nervous system. There is certainly no need for such elaborate tests as a computerized EEG or brain electrical activity mapping (BEAM): the American Academy of Neurology practice guidelines specifically state that ". . . the sensitivity and specificity [of these tests] fail to substantiate a role for these tests in the clinical diagnostic evaluation of individual patients for possible . . . attention deficit disorder."[42]

Similarly, tests of zinc levels and other trace elements are of no value in diagnosing ADHD, since ADHD reflects problems in the frontal lobes rather than deficiencies in these elements. This applies to tests for allergies and other substances, as well: while some ADHD children suffer from allergies, the identification and treatment of allergies usually has little or no bearing on symptoms of ADHD.

Evaluating the Adult with ADHD

In spite of the burgeoning interest in adult ADHD in the past decade, many professionals still consider evaluating an adult for ADHD to be a tricky undertaking.

In some respects, it is easier to interview adults about ADHD symptoms because they are generally more articulate and introspective than children. They know more about ADHD too: many request an evaluation after seeing a television program or reading a book on ADHD or after having had a child receive a diagnosis of ADHD.

In other respects, however, diagnosing ADHD in an adult is more difficult than making the diagnosis in a child. It is often difficult, for example, to obtain an accurate history of childhood symptoms, since human memory is so fallible. Dr. Paul Wender at the University of Utah has dealt with this problem by asking parents of his adult patients to complete the Conners Scale as they would have when the patient was a child. This approach can yield useful information but, again, we have to deal with the memory factor. The occasional patient can produce old report cards that attest to early problems: a sixty-two-year-old gentleman in my practice recently brought in report cards his mother had saved for over fifty years, and the teachers' comments from so long ago were big red flags for ADHD.

Rating Scales and Objective Measures

Diagnosis is complicated, too, by the fact that until recently we had no standards for judging just how impaired a person is in comparison with others his age. As subjective as rating scales for children are, at least now they have been standardized on large groups so that we can say with some confidence, "This child obtained a higher score on ratings of hyperactivity than ninety-five percent of children his age would be expected to obtain."

This problem has been tackled in slightly different ways by Dr. Tom Brown at Yale University and by Dr. Kevin Murphy at the University of Massachusetts. Dr. Brown's efforts have resulted in the Brown Attention and Activation Disorders Scale,[43] a questionnaire that asks people to rate themselves on a scale from 0 (no problem) to 3 (very much a problem) on forty items such as "Easily frustrated; excessively impatient" and "Procrastinates excessively; keeps putting things off." The scale can also be completed independently by a spouse or close friend to provide independent information about the person's problems in these areas.

Dr. Murphy has taken a different approach. As he has pointed out, the DSM-IV diagnostic criteria are based on field trials with children and adolescents, so we cannot assume that the criteria apply to adults as well. Dr. Murphy devised a checklist solely for adults based on the DSM-IV symptoms and administered the checklist to 720 adults in the general population.[44] The resulting information allows us to say with greater certainty whether an individual is more inattentive or hyperactive than others his age.

Continuous performance tests, described above, can also be of help in diagnosing ADHD in some adults. Unfortunately, the norms for adults are based on somewhat smaller groups than might be ideal but, even when performance on these tasks results in scores in the normal range, the effort that some adult patients have to expend to achieve this level of performance is a clear indication of problems.

Finding the Right Professional

If you've looked in the health section of your local newspaper lately, you might have noticed that many professionals are now advertising themselves as experts in the field of ADHD. Perhaps you have noticed, too, that ADHD clinics seem to be sprouting up like mushrooms after a rain. How do you know if these professionals are as good as they claim to be? And how do you know what kind of specialist you need? A psychiatrist? A psychologist? A developmental pediatrician? What's the difference between the various specialists and how do you go about finding the one who's right for you?

Briefly, the different professionals and their areas of expertise are as follows:

- *Psychiatrists* are physicians who have several years of specialty training in the diagnosis and treatment of so-called "mental disorders," including ADHD. All psychiatrists can prescribe medication; psychiatrists who specialize in prescribing medication are sometimes called "psychopharmacologists" to set them apart from other psychiatrists.
- *Psychologists* complete postgraduate training in the diagnosis and treatment of mental disorders, with an emphasis on how to conduct research on such disorders. They cannot prescribe medications because they do not have medical training, but they are trained to administer and interpret tests of intelligence, academic achievement, and personality.
- *Social workers* complete postgraduate training which prepares them to work in social service agencies and to provide therapy, in either an agency setting or private practice. In my experience, many social workers are excellent psychotherapists who can do an outstanding job of helping with the psychological issues that so many ADHD individuals face. Few, however, are specifically trained in diagnosis so, while they might suspect ADHD, they would not be able to make a diagnosis of ADHD with certainty.

As my colleague Dr. Sam Goldstein has so succinctly observed on more than one occasion, "The letters behind the name don't tell you who can play the game!'' While professional credentials may count in terms of insurance reimbursement, there is no guarantee that an advanced degree indicates knowledge and expertise in ADHD. Some psychiatrists and psychologists know a great deal about diagnosing and treating ADHD; some do not.

Since many ADHD children have coexisting psychiatric disorders, speech/language disorders, and learning disabilities, the professional who evaluates a child for ADHD must also have considerable knowledge in these related areas. For the most part, family practice physicians, pediatricians, neurologists, and family therapists have only minimal training and expertise in these areas, so coexisting conditions can be overlooked.

Finally, don't make the mistake of assuming that a nationally known expert can necessarily do a better job than a mental health professional who is closer to home. As I've traveled around the country conducting workshops on ADHD, I've been impressed with the caliber of professionals working in some very out-of-the-way places. It's generally preferable to work with a local professional, not just for the sake of convenience and cost, but because local professionals know about local resources. They usually know the professionals in the school system and in other service agencies and they are on the spot to help you put a treatment plan in place for your child.

The Cost of Care

Even when you find a professional with whom you would like to work, financial considerations might make engaging that professional very difficult. Under what is euphemistically called ''managed care,'' insurance companies have made it difficult for people who need mental health services to obtain them. If you belong to a health maintenance organization (HMO) in which all health care is provided by salaried professionals who work for the plan, you are limited to those professionals unless you pay for services yourself. In many cases, even obtaining an appointment with a mental health professional within ''the plan'' involves navigating a maze of advice nurses, pediatricians, and family practitioners, a process that can be arduous, time-consuming, and frustrating.

If you belong to a preferred provider organization (PPO), you will still be limited to obtaining services from professionals who are approved by that group and you will still have to go through the process of obtaining a referral to a mental health specialist. However, you might be able to recoup some of the cost of seeing a professional who is not a member of the PPO if you have chosen coverage that provides at least partial reimbursement for outside services.

Good mental health care is expensive—there's no getting around that. Skilled professionals expect to be compensated for their knowledge and their expertise. If your insurance won't help defray the costs of care, or if you haven't obtained satisfactory care within your insurance plan, what should you do?

Begin by determining how much of the cost of outside care your health plan will cover. If you are in a PPO and have chosen "high-option" coverage, your health plan will cover some of the cost of care from a professional outside of the PPO network. If you have not elected this coverage, or if you are in an HMO, try to locate an agency or a professional who will agree to work on a sliding fee scale. The school psychologist, guidance counselor, or principal may know of such an agency or individual. If not, you might contact your local mental health association or the local chapter of CH.A.D.D. or ADDA.

Be forewarned, however, that most top-flight professionals can't provide services at discounted rates. Many, however, are willing to work out a payment plan.

When the Diagnosis Is ADHD

When a credible professional confirms your suspicions of ADHD, you may feel a flood of emotions.

"When we learned that Mitchell had ADHD, my first reaction was 'Oh, no, that can't be true!' I thought kids with ADHD were completely out of control, totally wild. A little boy in Mitchell's class has ADHD and he's a monster! Mitchell isn't like that at all.

"My husband took it even harder than I did. At first, he was angry with the doctor, like it was the doctor's fault. I think one of the reasons it hit him so hard was because *he* was a hyperactive kid. He had a lot of problems growing up—nobody really understood ADHD when he was a kid—and I know he's afraid that Mitchell will have to go through what he went through. I think he feels guilty, too, like it's his fault for passing this on to his son."

Or, like some parents, you might feel relieved that someone has finally put a name to your child's problems.

"Cassie's been such a puzzle to us for so long. We could never understand why she just couldn't seem to follow the rules and get with the program. Jim always thought she was just spoiled and that if we—meaning me—would crack down on her, she would shape up.

"I'm really glad that we finally know what's going on with her. Of course, I'm not thrilled that my child has ADHD. But at least we can quit running in circles and start to get her the kind of help she needs."

Explaining ADHD to Children

Children, too, react in different ways to learning that they have ADHD. Some need to save face and steadfastly deny that they have any problems. Others—perhaps the majority—are as relieved as their parents to know that there's an explanation for their difficulties and that help is available.

How should we explain a diagnosis of ADHD in such a way that the child can understand his problems and yet not feel that he or she is seriously damaged or deficient or—what all children dread most—"different"? Ten years ago, I used the analogy of a car that was out of gas to explain ADHD. In their delightful book, *Putting on the Brakes,** Dr. Patricia Quinn and Judith Stern used the analogy of a bicycle with faulty brakes.

But these analogies, apt though they might be, are not altogether satisfactory because they still convey the message that the child is in some way broken or defective. As one of my young patients so poignantly phrased it, "My brain is messed up."

* New York: Magination Press, 1991.

Nor does telling children about eminent people who have had ADHD seem to help. Some ADHD youngsters do enjoy reading biographies of famous people who had problems similar to theirs—people like Thomas Edison and Winston Churchill—but not all children can take comfort from this knowledge. Indeed, as one of my young patients aptly observed, "Yeah, but they're famous and I'm not!"

Instead, I now tell my young ADHD patients that they may be the descendants of a long line of hunters, warriors, adventurers, and explorers, a line that stretches back two hundred thousand years to the beginnings of modern man. As I explain in *Distant Drums, Different Drummers*,* the book I wrote for young people with ADHD, their skills were very highly valued in years past; in fact, leaders in many societies, including our own, were drawn from their ranks. Now, however, the very qualities that made them successful for so many centuries make it hard for them to fit into a modern world run by less adventuresome people, whom author Thom Hartmann[45] describes as "farmers."

ADHD children—girls as well as boys—are usually enthusiastic about this explanation. Instead of seeing themselves as defective or damaged, they understand that certain aspects of their behavior, while not bad in themselves, bring them into conflict in today's world. Parents, too, like this explanation, because it reframes the condition in a positive light and removes the stigma of a "disorder," while at the same time setting the stage for change.

* Bethesda, Md.: Cape Publications, 1995.

CHAPTER 4

WHAT CAUSES ADHD?

Overview: Then and Now

Then: A decade ago, it was not uncommon for parents to be blamed for the problems of their ADHD children. Another popular belief at the time was that ADHD symptoms were caused by consumption of refined sugar and food additives. Additive-free diets such as the Feingold Diet were still in vogue, and many pediatricians recommended restricting the amount of sugar in the diets of their young patients with ADHD.

At the same time, however, evidence was mounting for a brain-behavior connection in ADHD. Breakthroughs in brain imaging technology offered the tantalizing possibility that we could actually identify the specific brain regions involved. The hope, of course, was that identification of these regions would lead to definitive diagnostic tests for ADHD, as well as to more effective treatments.

There was also an emerging awareness that ADHD tends to "run in families." Although some argued that this simply meant that troubled families can be expected to raise troubled children, others interpreted this as evidence for a genetic factor in ADHD.

Now: Although we do not yet have laboratory tests that can confirm a diagnosis of ADHD, much new knowledge has been gained in a decade.

Across the country, parents of ADHD children felt the weight of guilt and self-blame drop from their shoulders when Dr. Alan Zametkin's work indicating a physiological basis for ADHD was trumpeted on the front pages of *The New York Times* and *The Washington Post*.

On the genetic front, too, there has been impressive progress. As geneticists have availed themselves of advances in molecular biology to study the role of heredity in ADHD, it has become clear that ADHD is highly heritable. Most recently, they have identified some specific locations on certain genes that may play important roles in ADHD.

Are Parents to Blame?

If you are the parent of an ADHD child, you've surely gone through an anxious and confused period wondering "What is wrong with my child?" At some point you might have suspected environmental causes such as food allergies. Maybe you blamed a teacher or two: "His teacher is too impatient" or "He's bored in school because he's too bright for his current grade." Perhaps you attributed problems to traumatic events in the child's life—things like a move to a new area or the death of a close friend or relative.

Almost certainly you've been through the agony of self-blame, wondering what you did, or failed to do, that caused your child's problems. This is especially likely if there has been a divorce or if one parent suffers from depression, alcoholism, or another psychiatric disorder. In the past, at least, many mental health professionals, along with others in the community, were only too willing to join you in placing the blame on your shoulders.

In our society, it is widely assumed that child-rearing practices are the single most important factor in whether a child becomes a successful, well-adjusted adult or an unhappy failure. Many, if not most, people believe that babies are formless lumps of clay, waiting to be shaped and molded by their experiences, especially those that take place very early in life.

No one doubts that severely traumatic experiences such as abuse, neglect, or loss of a parent can have a profound effect on the developing child. No one doubts, either, the importance of stable, loving caretakers in the life of every child. However, the theory that good parenting is *the* determining factor in child adjustment is probably considerably overstated.

This idea dates back to Sigmund Freud, the father of psychoanalysis. Freud's followers in particular emphasized the importance of early experiences in forming adult personality and psychological adjustment. Behaviorists, too, whose work formed the basis for behavior modification, also viewed environmental factors such as parenting as the most important determinants of child behavior. Today, professionals trained in family therapy tell us that children's emotional and behavioral difficulties stem from disturbances in the way the family operates as a system, that is, the troublesome behavior of an ADHD child might reflect marital problems, say, or problems between a parent and a grandparent. Thus, once again there is the implication that parental problems cause disorders such as ADHD.

Is there evidence to support this theory? Dr. Russell Barkley, who has devoted a distinguished career to research with ADHD children and their families, doesn't think so. As he pointed out over a decade ago,[46] this theory cannot explain the high incidence of learning disabilities, minor physical anomalies, and frequent illnesses in infancy among ADHD children. Nor can this theory account for the fact that many parents of ADHD children have successfully raised other children who have no symptoms of ADHD.

It is true, as any parent of an ADHD child knows from experience, that parents treat an ADHD child differently from the way in which they treat the child's brothers and sisters. In fact, many of these parents say that they have always had to provide much closer supervision and control over the ADHD child, simply because his behavior demanded it. Many, too, feel bad about this.

"I know Conner thinks we pick on him and that we favor his sister. 'How come Little Miss Perfect never gets in trouble? How come it's always me getting yelled at and grounded?' He's right: I never have to raise my voice with Lindsey—but with Conner it seems like all I do is yell."

"All of the other children in the neighborhood are allowed to go to the pool by themselves at his age. But if I'm not right there to watch Aaron's every move, you can bet that he'll be sent home within ten minutes."

"All hell broke loose at our house when Joey found out that he's not going to get his learner's permit when he turns sixteen. The first thing he said was that we let his older brother and sister get their permits when they turned sixteen. And it's true; we did and we haven't had any cause to regret it. But Joey's a different story. We can't even trust him to take out the trash by himself, much less turn him loose behind the wheel of a car."

These differences are as obvious in the laboratory as they are in the home. In his lab, Dr. Barkley found that parents were more controlling and negative with their ADHD children than with their non-ADHD children. They issued more commands ("Come over here now") and prohibitions ("Don't play with that—leave it alone") and were less responsive to the ADHD child's bids for attention than to the same behavior in their other children. The children differed in behavior too: compared to their siblings, ADHD children were considerably more negative and disobedient.

From these findings, some researchers might have concluded that the parents were causing the problem, that the ADHD child's behavior was simply a response to negative and overcontrolling parent behavior. But Dr. Barkley took his research a step further and asked whether the parents' behavior might be at least partly a *response* to the ADHD child's difficult behavior rather than simply a cause. In a half-dozen well-executed studies, Dr. Barkley and his colleagues demonstrated convincingly that parent behavior is greatly influenced by child behavior. When, for example, the ADHD children were treated with stimulant medication, the same parents who were negative and controlling became more positive and responsive when the child's behavior improved as a result of medication.

In general, then, it seems safe to conclude that poor child-rearing practices do not *cause* ADHD but they certainly play a very significant role in determining outcome. This is especially true in the case of ADHD children with difficult temperaments, as we discuss in the following section.

Was He Born This Way?

From the discussion above, we can see that children actively help to shape their relationships with others through their own behavior. Babies are not simply blank slates upon which experience writes. Rather, parents have always known what research has only recently revealed: infants have individual personal styles, or *temperaments,* which may be obvious from the first months of life.

Some babies are placid and easygoing: when wet or hungry, they make their needs known with whimpers or quiet crying. Other babies are much more intense: if their needs are not met quickly, they burst into red-faced howls. Similarly, while some infants adapt readily to new experiences such as the first solid food or the first bath, others scream and protest vigorously when something new is introduced.

These patterns of temperament were originally investigated in the New York Longitudinal Study, a fascinating study that began forty years ago.[47] Under the direction of Doctors Stella Chess and Alexander Thomas, this investigation tracked a large group of children from birth through late adolescence. The findings, since corroborated by investigators in other cultures around the world, revealed that many children show distinctive temperaments that can be identified quite early in life. Although temperament is not very stable in the newborn period, stabilization begins in the early months of life and increases as the child enters the toddler years and early childhood.

Researchers have agreed on three major temperamental styles:

■ **Easy children** (who accounted for about forty percent of those in the original study group) are generally positive in mood and quick to smile. They adjust well to changes in schedules and accept new situations with little fuss. Their reactions tend to be mild or moderate in intensity and, when such a child creates a ruckus, it is a signal that something is indeed amiss.

- **Slow-to-warm-up children** dislike change. They react to new situations by quietly withdrawing. However, while they might appear shy in new situations, they gradually make a good adjustment if they are allowed to proceed at their own pace. These children accounted for about fifteen percent of the original study group.

- **Difficult children** (who comprised about ten percent of the original study group) have difficulty settling into a predictable routine. Their mood is generally negative and they react poorly to new situations, adapting only after many exposures to a new food or a new setting. Their reactions are often loud, forceful, and intense—screams instead of whimpers—and it may be difficult to soothe them or distract them from a bad mood or a forbidden activity.

Raising a temperamentally difficult child can be a challenge even for experienced, confident parents. Parents who have coped with these children admit that they can drive even the most patient of parents to the brink of despair. What happens to these children as they grow?

Temperament and Psychiatric Disorders

Is there a relationship between early "difficult" temperament and psychiatric disorders? There certainly appears to be: in the original study group, seventy percent of those with a difficult temperament developed some type of behavior disorder in childhood![48] Subsequent studies have supported these findings: in Quebec, for example, Dr. Michel Maziade found that of the nine to ten percent of children in the population who comprise the group with the most difficult temperament, about one in two develops a clinical disorder in childhood.[49]

What kinds of problems do "difficult" children develop? A decade ago, researchers linked a difficult temperament with ADHD, as I noted in *Your Hyperactive Child*. More recent evidence, however, such as that from Dr. Maziade's group, indicates that a difficult temperament, similar to that described in the original New York Longitudinal Study, actually predicts oppositional defiant disorder rather than ADHD. As noted in

Chapter 2, Dr. Maziade found that ODD is often diagnosed in children whose early temperament was characterized by a tendency to withdraw in the face of new situations; poor adaptability to change; predominantly negative mood; intense emotional reactions; and low distractibility (a tendency to "get stuck" in an activity, a course of action, or a bad mood).*

How strong is the influence of adverse temperament on the later development of psychiatric disorders? A difficult temperament puts a child at significant risk for such disorders, but researchers agree that temperament is just one factor in a complicated equation. Other factors, such as family dysfunction, marital problems, and inconsistent discipline also play critical roles. In fact, in Dr. Maziade's large-scale studies, *most* of the difficult children who lived in dysfunctional families developed oppositional disorders. In contrast, *almost none* of the difficult children who lived in families with generally high levels of functioning developed disorders. In particular, even very difficult children were apt to do well in families in which parents made the rules quite clear, agreed with each other about the rules, and were consistent in enforcing them.

Could Something Have Damaged His Brain?

In keeping with the idea of "minimal brain damage" popular in the 1950s and 1960s, early researchers looked to the nine months before birth (prenatal period) or to the birth process itself (perinatal period) for clues about what causes ADHD. Others explored damage to the developing brain after birth, caused by exposure to toxic substances (lead, for example), or by an ongoing allergic reaction to certain chemicals and food additives. These lines of inquiry attracted considerable interest, but for the majority of ADHD children they have proved to be blind alleys.

---

* Note that low persistence/attention span and high activity level do *not* characterize this group: instead, Dr. Maziade found that these traits were more likely to be associated with developmental delays.

Prenatal and Perinatal Problems

Research conducted in the 1970s and 1980s[50] showed that mothers of ADHD children were more likely than mothers of non-ADHD children to be under the age of twenty when the child was born. They were also more likely to report poor health during pregnancy, as well as toxemia (an infection that results in bacterial toxins in the bloodstream) and eclampsia (coma or convulsions with high blood pressure, fluid retention, and abnormal proteins in the urine). In addition, labor lasting more than thirteen hours and fetal distress were more common in the ADHD group. More recent research has uncovered a link between complications during pregnancy (e.g., accident, illness, bleeding, excessive nausea, weight loss, or excessive weight gain) or delivery and ADHD that is strongest for ADHD children with comorbid problems but without a family history of ADHD.[51]

Recent research also indicates that premature babies who are very premature (less than thirty-two weeks) and premature babies who are small for gestational age—that is, they weigh less than we would expect, given the time since conception—are more likely to have a short attention span in childhood.[52] Babies who are particularly low in weight are also at increased risk for motor problems and learning disabilities.

Other investigators have found a connection between ADHD and maternal alcohol use, drug use, and smoking during pregnancy. Since people who abuse one of these substances are likely to abuse others, it is difficult to sort out the effects of a single substance. Nevertheless, alcohol abuse during pregnancy is clearly linked to attentional, learning, and behavioral problems in children, as seen in children with fetal alcohol syndrome and fetal alcohol effects.[53] The effects of smoking during pregnancy are clear too: there is a strong link between maternal smoking during pregnancy and ADHD in their children.[54] It may be that exposure in utero to nicotine effects the dopamine system, a system known to be involved in ADHD. It may also be the case that since nicotine improves symptoms of adult ADHD, expectant ADHD mothers are more likely than others to find it more difficult to stop smoking during pregnancy.[55]

The effects of prenatal exposure to cocaine are also well known: compelling evidence points to the devastating effects of exposure to cocaine on the developing fetus. Children whose mothers used cocaine during pregnancy suffer a horrifying array of neurological, behavioral, intellectual, and emotional problems.[56]

In summary, there is a group of ADHD children whose problems probably stem at least in part from damage incurred before or during birth. These children, however, account for only a small percentage of those who are diagnosed with ADHD and they may be more likely to have comorbid problems.

Environmental Toxins

Pollutants and Toxic Substances. Following birth, damage to the developing brain can occur from exposure to hazardous substances such as asbestos, foam insulation, toxic waste products in the water supply, and pollutants in the air. The effects of one toxic substance, lead, have long been known: in addition to fatigue, pallor, irritability, nausea, and loss of appetite, lead poisoning can cause neurological damage and psychological problems.

In one recent study, for example, high levels of lead in the bone (a measure of cumulative lead exposure) were associated with an array of problems, including physical complaints, depression, attention problems, and aggression.[57] It doesn't take high levels of lead to cause problems: even low to moderate levels of lead can cause learning and attentional deficits. Nor are children who live in old tenements with peeling paint the only ones at risk, since even children who live in affluent areas can be exposed to lead when old water mains are disturbed during construction and from old paint removed during renovation projects. Thus, while it is unlikely that lead is the source of the problem for most ADHD children, we need to do all we can to protect our children from exposure to this and other toxins.

Medications and Allergic Substances. There is also convincing evidence that, for a small group of children, exposure to the anticonvulsant medication phenobarbital can produce hyperactivity. Even after medication is discontinued, symptoms of hyperactivity may remain.[58]

Other substances have also been implicated in ADHD. Food additives and preservatives, in particular, have been suspect since Dr. Benjamin

Feingold suggested that allergiclike reactions to these substances cause about half of all cases of ADHD. In addition to synthetic dyes and flavorings, Dr. Feingold believed that salicylates, found in aspirin and in many fruits and vegetables, also cause behavioral disturbances in some children.

Recently, enthusiasm for the Feingold Diet has been replaced by a concern about allergies to specific foods as a cause for ADHD. Dr. Doris Rapp, a pediatric allergist, is one of the better known advocates of dietary modification as a treatment for learning and behavior problems. However, as my coauthor Dr. Sam Goldstein and I pointed out in a previous book,* Dr. Rapp's claims and methods lack scientific backing and are considered questionable by the scientific community in general and by pediatric allergists in particular.

Finally, there are those who claim that refined sugar causes ADHD and a host of other ills as well. The "sugar-as-poison" notion was championed early on by Dr. Lendon Smith in books like *Improving Your Child's Behavior Chemistry* and *Feed Your Kids Right*. Pediatricians apparently found this idea appealing, as a 1983 survey indicated that almost half of the pediatricians surveyed sometimes recommended low-sugar diets for their patients with behavioral and attentional problems.[59]

From a more scientific perspective, however, it appears that refined sugar plays a negligible role in attention and behavior problems. In fact, study after study has shown that sugar has little impact on children's behavior, and experts such as Dr. Keith Conners flatly state that research findings do *not* justify eliminating sugar in the diets of ADHD children.[60]

Is It Hereditary?

As I reported a decade ago, parents of ADHD children are likely to describe their youngsters as "a chip off the old block." Parents of these children can often identify similar qualities in themselves, their mates, and members of the extended family. "He's just like me when I was his age," parents tell me. And, "His father is the sweetest man alive, but he makes

---

* *Attention Deficit Disorder and Learning Disabilities: Realities, Myths and Controversial Treatments.* New York: Doubleday, 1993.

me crazy because he can't remember anything from one minute to the next."

"I've done some reading and I'm sure that Michael's problems can be traced way back in our family. My father was pretty wild in his younger days. He did crazy stunts on motorcycles, fought with the bosses in the yard at the railroad, swam across the Allegheny River on a bet—all kinds of stories. He was a good worker but a hothead and a hell-raiser. He settled down a lot as he got older but he never was one to sit for very long. I didn't know his father because he died when I was a baby, but from everything I've heard about him, he was a wild man in his day, too."

Does ADHD "run in families," like diabetes and other conditions that have a genetic component? For many ADHD youngsters, this certainly seems to be the case: in comparison with other children, ADHD children are up to five times more likely to have a close family member who has ADHD. It is estimated that anywhere from eleven to thirty-eight percent of ADHD children have mothers who have ADHD and seventeen to forty-four percent have fathers who have ADHD. The familial component appears particularly strong in cases in which ADHD persists into the adult years: a parent with adult ADHD has about an eighty-four percent chance of having at least one ADHD child and a fifty-two percent chance of having two or more ADHD children.[61] Siblings are at risk too: siblings of ADHD children are three to four times more likely to have ADHD than siblings of non-ADHD children.[62]

Does this mean that ADHD is inherited? Or does it just mean that the ADHD child's difficulties are due to the stress of growing up in a rather chaotic environment? Studies of twin pairs in which one twin has ADHD can throw some light on the subject: among identical twins, who are genetically identical, we find that in the majority of cases, when one twin has ADHD, so does the other twin.[63,64] This rate drops significantly in fraternal twins, who, like twins, share a common environment but, like nontwin siblings, share only half of their genes with each other. Thus, these findings support a strong genetic component in ADHD.

Also, when we look at studies of adopted ADHD children, there appears to be a higher-than-average incidence of ADHD and related disorders among biological parents and other blood relatives, but a lower-than-average incidence of these problems in adoptive parents (who are carefully screened during the adoptive process).[65,66] From this, it appears that heredity has a stronger influence on ADHD than does environment.

Genetic factors might also help explain the increase in the number of people diagnosed with ADHD in recent years. For example, assortative mating—the tendency for people to select mates who are like themselves—could lead in many cases to families with a particularly heavy genetic "loading" for ADHD. Children in these families would be at particularly high risk for ADHD since, as a colleague of mine once observed, "You don't breed Great Danes and get Chihuahuas."

There is also the phenomenon that geneticists refer to as "anticipation," that is, the tendency for inherited disorders to show up earlier and/or with more severe symptoms in each successive generation. This happens because the genes responsible for the disorder actually expand as unstable strands of DNA known as "triplet repeats" increase in number from one generation to the next. Long known to occur in certain neuro-muscular disorders, anticipation has recently been found to occur in psychiatric disorders such as bipolar disorder and schizophrenia as well.[67,68] To date, there have been no published reports of anticipation in ADHD. In my clinical experience, however, I have seen so many cases in which symptoms of ADHD seemed to appear at an earlier age and with greater severity as ADHD is passed down from one generation to the next, so it would not be surprising if anticipation were found to occur in ADHD.

Finally, new research indicates that several genes responsible for regulation and function of the immune system have a strong association with ADHD. At Utah State University, researchers have found that many ADHD children and their parents have a defect in certain genes that play an important role in defending against infections. This defect, which was found in about fifty-five percent of ADHD subjects but in only eight percent of non-ADHD subjects, results in lower than normal concentrations of the complement C4B protein, a blood protein that plays an important role in defending against infections.[69,70] Researchers do not yet know whether a low level of C4B is merely a "marker" for ADHD (one that would explain why young ADHD children are so susceptible to chronic ear infections, for example) or whether low levels of maternal C4B during pregnancy might make them vulnerable to infections that could damage the developing brain of the fetus.

In summary, although not all cases of ADHD involve heredity, the evidence points to the role of genetic factors in the majority of cases. But what is it that the ADHD child inherits? Exciting research on the brain and behavior, discussed in the following section, suggests some answers to this question.

The Brain and Behavior

As the older terms "minimal brain damage" and "minimal brain dysfunction" suggest, scientists have long suspected brain malfunction as the cause of ADHD. Greatest interest has been focused on the part of the frontal lobes known as the prefrontal cortex, an area involved in the so-called "executive functions" of regulating attention and activity, inhibiting impulsive responding, planning ahead, and organizing time and space.

In spite of an avalanche of research, advances in our knowledge have come only slowly. Progress has been hindered by the incredible complexity and delicacy of the brain itself, and it is only recently that technology has helped scientists begin to unlock the mysteries of how the brain functions in conditions such as ADHD. To understand the difficulties faced by those who study the brain, it is helpful to know a bit about the brain and how it works.

The Brain: Pieces of the Puzzle

The brain consists of billions of nerve cells, each of which has hundreds of connections with other nerve cells. Groups of cells form highly specialized control centers, and fibers extending from these centers form pathways throughout the brain, linking the control centers with each other.

Each nerve cell consists of a cell body and a long projection called the axon. When a nerve cell fires, the message travels along the axon by electrical conduction. When the electrical impulse reaches the end of the axon, storage sacs there release a substance called a neurotransmitter. This substance crosses the tiny space between the axon and the next cell, where it excites a receptor and causes that cell to fire in turn.

After the message has been transmitted, the neurotransmitter must be removed or it would continue to send the same message forever. One method of removal is "reuptake": the neurotransmitter is taken back into the storage sacs in the sending cell. Another means of removal is through chemical breakdown and deactivation.

Since psychiatric disorders appear to result from problems in neurotransmitter systems, it is logical to treat these disorders with medications that correct the underlying chemical imbalances. Some of these medications increase the production of specific neurotransmitters or mimic the action of natural neurotransmitters. Others prevent reuptake of the neurotransmitter into storage sacs. In both cases, the result is a net increase in the amount of active neurotransmitter at the receptor site. Still other medications influence the sensitivity of particular receptors, making them more or less responsive to incoming messages.

The Brain and ADHD

Brain Structure. Just ten years ago, in *Your Hyperactive Child,* I wrote "[T]he basic structure of the brain in the hyperactive child appears to be intact—there are no obvious malformations or missing parts." Since then, however, new evidence has appeared that indicates that there are, indeed, differences in brain anatomy in ADHD children.

Using new magnetic resonance imaging (MRI) techniques which permit them to observe brain structures with increased clarity, neuroscientists at the National Institute of Mental Health and elsewhere have found structural differences in the brains of children with ADHD. Specifically, they have found that certain structures in the right prefrontal region of the brain are smaller in ADHD individuals than in non-ADHD individuals.[71] These structures and the circuits that connect them form the brain's "braking mechanism." Underactivity in this part of the brain could result in impulsive behavior and inability of an ADHD individual to "put on the brakes" in terms of controlling his own behavior.

Interestingly, maturation in these circuits continues into the third decade of life. Thus, as Dr. Xavier Castellanos at NIMH points out, delays in maturation of this region of the brain could account for the fact that many ADHD youngsters show progressive improvement in symptoms as they enter their thirties and forties.[72]

The Brain at Work. Some early studies of brain function in ADHD used electroencephalography (EEG) to measure the electrical activity that occurs when messages are transmitted from one brain cell to another. Because the EEG summarizes the electrical activity of millions of nerve cells, it is a rather crude technique for examining the brain at work. It's not surprising, then, that these early studies did not yield a great deal of information about brain function in ADHD.

More recently, neuroscientists have used sophisticated computer analyses of EEG patterns to "map" patterns of brain electrical activity associated with ADHD. This technique, known as *brain electrical activity mapping,* has revealed some intriguing differences in the patterns of brain electrical activity in ADHD and non-ADHD individuals. Specifically, differences have been found in right- versus left-brain activity and in electrical activity that occurs in response to a signal (such as a tone). These differences have been found in ADHD children with and without hyperactivity.[73]

The techniques of brain imaging have also provided us with a window into the working brain. Over a decade ago, scientists in Denmark used radioactive tracer substances to measure blood flow in different regions of the brain and found reduced blood flow in the frontal lobes in every ADHD child they examined. When these children were treated with stimulant medication, all showed increased blood flow in the affected areas.[74]

In the United States, Dr. Alan Zametkin and his colleagues at the National Institute of Mental Health used positron emission tomography (PET) scans to study the brain activity in adults with ADHD. This technique, which uses a radioactive tracer substance to study glucose metabolism in the brain, revealed reduced metabolic activity in brains of ADHD individuals. These reductions were most pronounced in the frontal and prefrontal regions and improved when stimulant medication was given.[75]

Chemical Messengers. Ten years ago, I was skeptical that we would soon learn much about the neurotransmitters involved in ADHD, given the great difficulties in studying these substances in living humans. And again, dedicated scientists proved my dour prediction wrong.

Although other neurotransmitters such as norepinephrine are also believed to play a role in ADHD, the neurotransmitter most closely linked with ADHD is dopamine. Dopamine is important in the regulation of motor activity, as we have long known from studies of patients with Parkinson's disease. In young children, who are almost constantly engaged in exploring their environment, dopamine levels are high. These levels drop quickly over the next dozen years *except* in children with ADHD: as the work of Dr. Xavier Castellanos and his colleagues at NIMH has shown, ADHD children have higher than normal levels of a breakdown product called homovanillic acid, which results from dopamine metabolism.[76] Not only were the highest levels of this acid found in the most hyperactive children: higher levels also predicted a better response to treatment with stimulants.

Other scientists have reason to suspect that dopamine plays a role in the personality trait called "novelty-seeking," a trait that includes impulsivity, excitability, hotheadedness, and changeability.[77] This, of course, sounds a lot like ADHD and, in fact, the same genetically mediated differences in dopamine transmission that seem to occur in individuals high in novelty-seeking have also been found by at least one group of researchers to occur in ADHD individuals.[78] Might this be one of the ways in which ADHD traits are passed along from generation to generation? It's still too early to tell, but it's clear that answers lie in the not-too-distant future.

Evolution and the Brain

As we see, scientists have documented differences in brain structure and function in people with and without ADHD. What should we make of these findings? Do these differences mean that people with ADHD are defective or deficient? Does it mean that they have a disorder or a disease?

When ADHD is accompanied by coexisting conditions such as depression, oppositional defiant disorder, conduct disorder, or an anxiety disorder, there is no question that the child suffers pain and causes problems for himself and for those around him. In such cases, it's obvious that we should consider the child as suffering from a disorder and make provisions for appropriate treatment.

But how about what I've come to think of as "garden variety" ADHD, that is, ADHD without any coexisting learning problems or psychiatric disorders? Certainly, ADHD individuals have difficulty meeting the demands they encounter as children—demands to sit still, pay attention, and organize themselves according to a relentless clock and calendar. But research, along with my own clinical experience, clearly shows that the prognosis for these youngsters is generally quite good; in fact, as adults, many go on to become highly successful, especially in professions and work settings in which their energy and willingness to take risks are considered advantages. For example, one study found that ADHD individuals have a bent for entrepreneurship, as indicated by the fact that almost four times as many adults diagnosed with ADHD owned their own businesses as did adults in a non-ADHD comparison group.[79] And—while I don't have scientific data to support this notion—have you ever met a firefighter or emergency room physician who could be described as phlegmatic, low-energy, or excessively cautious?

I think, then, that we might look upon ADHD as an evolutionary variant, a brain that Mother Nature designed to maximize the odds that Homo sapiens would survive in a world that needed impulsive individuals who wouldn't hesitate to jump in feetfirst when a situation demanded prompt action and quick reflexes. And I don't find it surprising that so many human societies have elevated these individuals to positions of leadership: think of Alexander the Great or, closer to our own time and place, think of warrior-leaders like George Washington or Dwight Eisenhower.

Until recently, I thought I was alone in viewing ADHD from this perspective. I was pleased, therefore, when my colleague and coauthor Sam Goldstein, in his book *Hyperactivity: Why Won't My Child Pay Attention*★ described these children as "risk-takers." I was even more excited to learn of Thom Hartmann's book, in which he described the ADHD individual as a hunter constrained to live in a world of farmers. More recently, I've been deeply gratified to see that renowned scientists like Dr. Russell Barkley, Dr. John Werry, and Dr. Peter Jensen agree that as Dr. Barkley states, "ADHD may simply represent a human trait and not a pathological condition in most cases."[80]

Dr. Werry, a pioneer in ADHD research, has been a proponent of this view for many years. Never one to mince words, Dr. Werry long ago described ADHD as "a biological variant made manifest by the affluent

★ New York: John Wiley, 1992.

society's insistence on universal literacy and its acquisition in a sedentary position." As Dr. Werry reminds us, while ADHD can be quite disabling in our literate society, this is not always the case: as scientists and clinicians who work with ADHD children must remember, we only see the ones with problems![81]

At the National Institute of Mental Health, Dr. Peter Jensen, chief of the Child and Adolescent Disorders Research Branch, believes that an evolutionary perspective can be applied to ADHD. Concerning hyperactivity, for example, he points out that high levels of activity would have been useful in a hunter-gatherer society to assist in foraging and spotting new opportunities, while rapidly shifting attention would have increased the individual's ability to scan the environment for potential resources or dangers. Impulsivity, too, would be adaptive in a primitive environment in which the individual had to pounce quickly on prey or dodge a predator.[82]

I do not intend to minimize or make light of the very real problems all ADHD individuals—children, adolescents, and adults—face in daily life in our Western world. In a society obsessed with academic achievement and with strict adherence to deadlines, ADHD individuals are indeed handicapped. Further, it is quite appropriate to provide accommodations for the difficulties ADHD causes them in school and in the workplace.

However, I think it's very important for ADHD children, many of whom have been drowning in negative feedback, to begin to see themselves and their characteristics in a more positive light. We must be careful that, in trying to help ADHD individuals with the problems they encounter, we don't overlook the fact that they also have many wonderful and valuable qualities. I for one would find a world of all farmers and no hunters a dull and colorless world indeed.

CHAPTER 5

MEDICAL TREATMENT OF ADHD

What Have We Learned in a Decade?

Overview: Then and Now

Then: A decade ago, medication was often considered the treatment of last resort for ADHD, and many experts advised parents to exhaust all other treatments before turning to medication. Stimulant medication— particularly Ritalin—was virtually the only medication prescribed, although there were indications that tricylic antidepressants were a good "second line" when stimulants failed, and that other medicines such as clonidine might also be of help in ADHD.

It was just over a decade ago, too, that the Church of Scientology began a self-serving campaign against the use of medication for ADHD children. This brief but vicious campaign left a legacy of misinformation about stimulant medication with which parents and professionals must still contend.

Now: Medication is now recognized as the first line of treatment for both children and adults with ADHD and the emerging consensus is that medication should be employed sooner rather than later. Stimulants are still the treatment of choice for uncomplicated ADHD, but our knowledge about who is most likely to benefit from these medications has increased considerably.

So, too, has the array of medications available. Along with a new stimulant (Adderal), a variety of medications have found a place in the treatment of ADHD. More precise diagnostic practices now enable us to be more precise in tailoring specific treatments to specific symptoms, resulting in greatly improved functioning for many children with ADHD.

There are still many myths and misconceptions about medication, particularly stimulant medication. Periodically, media coverage contributes to these misconceptions and fuels parental fears. Even when an article or broadcast treats the subject in an evenhanded and objective fashion, editors can't seem to resist sensational headlines, like "Ritalin: Are We Overmedicating Our Kids?" (*Newsweek,* March 18, 1996) and "Children's Cure or Adults' Crutch?" (*The Washington Post,* April 11, 1995).

Nevertheless, the general population seems much better informed now about ADHD and the medications used to treat it. As public awareness of ADHD has grown, the use of medication as part of a treatment regimen has gained greater acceptance.

Stimulant Medication

More than half a century ago, Dr. Charles Bradley reported that central nervous system stimulants had the unexpected effect of calming restless, hyperactive children. Dr. Bradley's findings were generally ignored until the 1950s, when the development of new medications for treating psychiatric disorders led to renewed interest in stimulant medication.

Today, mental health professionals consider medication to be the most effective form of treatment for ADHD. Certainly, with an estimated three to four percent of youths in the U.S. receiving stimulant medication,[83] it is the most common form of treatment for this condition.

Stimulants used to treat ADHD are:

- Ritalin (methylphenidate)*
- Dexedrine (dextroamphetamine)

* On first mentioning a medication, I will follow the medical convention of giving the brand name, followed (in parentheses) by the generic equivalent. Thereafter, I will use whichever name seems to be more commonly recognized.

- Cylert (pemoline)
- Adderal (a mixture of four amphetamine salts).

Ritalin is by far the most commonly prescribed stimulant, not because it is necessarily better than the other stimulants, but because physicians preferred to prescribe it after Dexedrine gained a bad image as "speed." Ritalin and Dexedrine are both available in long-acting forms and, although research indicates that the long-acting forms of both are effective, many clinicians believe that the long-acting form of Dexedrine is more effective and better tolerated than the long-acting form of Ritalin.

Cylert has never been in widespread use for a number of reasons, including the fact that it requires several days to several weeks before effects are observable. In December 1996, following the reports of several cases of acute liver failure, the Food and Drug Administration issued a warning and Cylert is no longer considered a first-line drug therapy for ADHD.

Adderal, a combination of four amphetamine salts, was used in the past for weight control. Recently it has been introduced for the treatment of ADHD and, in a study comparing it with Ritalin, it was rated as superior to Ritalin in terms of both symptom control and side effects.[84] More studies are needed, but Adderal looks like an extremely promising treatment for many children and adults with ADHD.

How Does Stimulant Medication Work?

Stimulant medication helps the ADHD child focus his attention and control his activity level. It also helps him regulate his behavior so that it is less impulsive, disorganized, and chaotic. Exactly *how* stimulants do this is still a matter of much conjecture among scientists, although there is general agreement that they primarily affect the neurotransmitter dopamine and, to a lesser extent, norepinephrine: the fact is, that is what they do— *and they do it for more than ninety percent of children with uncomplicated ADHD.*[85]

Benefits of Medication

When stimulant medication is effective, improvement is immediate and sometimes quite dramatic. What can you expect to see?

Reductions in Hyperactive, Impulsive Behavior. Children on medication are not less active across the board: in active, boisterous play situations, they dash about like other children. In settings that call for more restrained behavior, however, they are better able to sit without fidgeting and jumping around.

Improved self-control means that your child is more likely to resist temptation and that he can obey rules that were frequently violated in the past—rules like "Don't touch things in stores" and "Don't interrupt when others are talking." The child who previously shoved his way to the head of the line can await his turn and the youngster who was antsy and obnoxious at the table after finishing his meal can now sit while others finish theirs.

In school, the child no longer calls out or plunges into his work before waiting for instructions. Work is completed more carefully and neatly, as opposed to the child's previous slapdash, messy productions.

When his doctor recommended a trial of Ritalin, the parents of nine-year-old Todd were initially skeptical. Somewhat reluctantly, they agreed on a two-week trial of medication.

Two weeks later, they returned to the doctor, bringing with them a sheaf of notes. "You know that we had a lot of reservations about the medicine," Todd's mother stated. "But he certainly seems a lot calmer now. In fact, he actually sat through services at church for two Sundays in a row without a major scene."

"And on that trip we took last weekend—he wasn't all over the car, giving me fits," Todd's father chimed in.

Todd's teacher also noticed a big change, they added. Todd was able to sit and complete his work without constant trips to the bathroom, the pencil sharpener, or the teacher's desk. Even the bus driver saw an improvement: "He thought Todd must be coming down with the flu because he didn't have to yell at him for bouncing on the seats or jumping in the aisles."

praise

Criticism

if Chad gets only faces
Monday - Thursday Fridays
maybe he could have a
privilege such as computer or
working w/ special art materials etc

Teacher →

If alot more criticism
Put 10 pennies in your pocket and transfer one
to the other pocket everytime you praise your child
promise any not to say a critical word until
you've put all 10 pennies from one pocket to the other

"Work before you play"
Time out in chair anywhere
explain why 6"iving" time out !!!

— 1 day is good for taking away something —

Book Dr Russell Barkleys book "Taking Charge of
ADHD.

Improved Attention and Organization. You can also expect your child to be less distractible, absentminded, and disorganized. His teacher might report that he now pays attention to his work instead of gazing out the window, fiddling with his pencil, or chatting with others. Thus, there is less unfinished work sent home to be completed.

You may also notice that your child no longer needs to have instructions repeated several times: because he is better able to focus his attention, he is more likely to absorb the information the first time around.

Better Tolerance for Frustration. Stimulant medication also helps with aggression and poor frustration tolerance. You may notice that your child is better able to cope with disappointment and less likely to burst into angry tears when he is thwarted in any way. As one parent observed of her child, "He doesn't fall apart over little things any more and he doesn't go wild if he doesn't get his own way."

Improved Relationships with Peers, Family. Years ago, Dr. Russell Barkley reported immediate reductions in parent-child conflict as a result of stimulant medication. Teacher-child relationships improve too: teachers reduce their negative feedback as the child's behavior and academic performance improve. Although some ADHD children continue to have social problems, many get along better with friends and classmates as their bossy and impulsive behavior decreases. Even sibling squabbles may diminish because, with medication, the ADHD child is no longer as annoying or as aggressive toward brothers and sisters.

Improvements in Language. The organizing effects of stimulant medication also extend to the domain of receptive and expressive language. Ritalin, for example, has been found to improve auditory attention and auditory processing in ADHD children.[86] Improvements in conversational skills have also been reported with stimulants: in Toronto, Dr. Rosemary Tannock and her associates found that ADHD children treated with Ritalin were less likely to initiate conversations at inappropriate times and more likely to respond appropriately in conversation, such as when asked a question.[87]

Enhanced Academic Achievement. Some critics have charged that stimulant medication produces improvements in behavior at the expense of the child's ability to learn. Recent research, however, indicates that stimulants actually *improve* cognitive function and memory in ADHD children.[88] For many ADHD children, treatment with stimulant medication results in significant improvement in reading, spelling, and arithmetic. The amount of work completed increases, while errors decrease.[89] In one study, for example, medication resulted in a thirty percent increase in the number of arithmetic problems completed, with no loss in accuracy.[90] In another study, researchers reported a twenty-five percent improvement in spelling tasks as a result of medication.[91] Improvements in handwriting, when they occur, are sometimes dramatic: a child whose written work formerly looked like a battle between two drunk chickens can now produce a legible manuscript.

Not all children whose classroom behavior improves on medication show corresponding gains in academic skills and performance. This is not surprising, since medication cannot substitute for appropriate remedial intervention if a child is far behind academically due to unidentified learning disabilities. In such children, however, a combination of remedial help and stimulant medication produces much better results than either intervention alone.[92]

Better Self-Esteem. With improvement across so many areas, can we expect corresponding changes in self-esteem? That is, in fact, what we see in the majority of ADHD children for whom stimulant medication is effective. Although a few children resist taking medication because they believe it means they are in some way inferior or defective, most children who benefit from stimulant medication also report that they like themselves better when they are on medication.[93]

Side Effects

Short-Term Side Effects. Side effects of stimulant medication usually occur at the start of treatment, are mild in nature, and diminish rapidly. To minimize side effects, the child should be started at the lowest dose (5 milligrams of Ritalin or Dexedrine for children seven and older; 2.5 milligrams of Ritalin or Dexedrine for those age six and under).

The most common side effects of stimulant medication are poor appetite and insomnia. To minimize appetite problems, give medication twenty to thirty minutes after meals. (Note: Give medication with water, not milk or orange juice.) Also, feed your child protein at breakfast: research indicates that a protein-based breakfast helps improve performance throughout the day. There is no divine decree that turkey sandwiches, hot dogs, or chicken nuggets can't be eaten at breakfast, so you have lots of options. Try toasted ham and cheese on an English muffin or reheated pizza, along with a glass of milk, to get some protein into your ADHD child in the morning. For the occasional child who isn't hungry at dinner, a bedtime milk shake made with ice cream and a liquid dietary supplement will keep the child well nourished.

Insomnia is a bit trickier to deal with. Suggestions for helping ADHD children with sleep problems are outlined in Chapter 7.

Headaches, stomachaches, and dizziness can appear as side effects of medication if the child is started on a higher dose without being stepped up gradually. These symptoms can also appear in some youngsters who receive two or three doses per day; since there is some overlap across doses, there may be periods when the child receives an effective dose higher than the one intended.[94] For many ADHD children, this is not problematic, but you should be alert to this possibility.

At the start of treatment, your child might become a bit difficult and fussy for about twenty minutes when medication wears off. This effect, known as "rebound," tends to be more pronounced in younger children but usually diminishes rather quickly when it is mild in nature. If the child falls apart or becomes extremely active and unmanageable when medication wears off, this is an indication that the medication or the dose may not be the right one for the child.

Long-Term Side Effects. This is what parents fear most—that a medication used to treat today's problem will result in more serious problems in the future. It's reassuring to know that stimulants do not produce lasting changes in heart rate or blood pressure[95] and that no studies have reported adverse long-term side effects of stimulant medication.

Prescribing and Monitoring Medication

As one would expect, most pediatricians today are familiar enough with stimulants to do a perfectly competent job in uncomplicated cases of ADHD. In complicated cases, however (for example, if comorbidity is involved, or if the child has a poor response to stimulants), a child psychiatrist who specializes in psychopharmacology should prescribe and monitor medication.

Beginning Treatment. Prescribing practices have changed over the years. Stimulant doses are no longer calculated on the basis of body weight, as was the case ten years ago, when I wrote *Your Hyperactive Child,* because there seems to be no correlation between body weight and effective dose.[96] Instead, current practice is to prescribe low doses and to move forward from there, monitoring the child's response carefully along the way.

For a child age seven or older, it is common practice to begin with 5 milligrams of Ritalin or Dexedrine in the morning and at noon and to increase each dose by 5 milligrams at weekly intervals until a good response is observed.* This process should be monitored closely by a professional. However, noted child psychiatrist Dr. Harold Eist recommends beginning with 5 milligrams of Ritalin or Dexedrine in the morning for three days. A second dose can then be added and, after three days, a third dose can be added. If you don't see benefits or side effects, the physician might increase the dose to 10 milligrams in the morning, after which the noon dose and the late-day dose can be added at three-day intervals.

During this period, you and your child's teacher should observe the child closely. (Rating scales, described in Chapter 3, are helpful for this purpose.) Even if your child's behavior isn't troublesome at home, it's a good idea to give medication on weekends as well as on schooldays initially and to make all changes in dose on weekends, so you can observe the results.

Include your child in the monitoring process too. Although ADHD children are notorious for lack of insight into their behavior, even young children can see a difference in their behavior on stimulant medication, if only to note that "My teacher doesn't yell at me as much" or "I don't have so many time-outs now." Children should also be questioned about side effects, too, because they sometimes report side effects such as drowsiness or dizziness that parents do not observe.[97]

Although some doctors begin treatment with long-acting (sustained release) medication, I don't agree with this practice. Because children vary in their response to long-acting stimulants, this makes it very difficult to determine the most helpful dose and timing of medication. I also don't recommend the use of generic stimulants, because some children

---

* With younger children, the starting dose should be 2.5 milligrams and dose increments should also be 2.5 milligrams.

have variable and unpredictable responses to them.[98] While you are determining the correct dose of medication for your child, avoid both generic and long-acting forms of stimulant medication.

If an initial trial of stimulant medication isn't helpful or if your child complains of side effects, don't be too quick to conclude that medication is not effective. Research and clinical experience indicate that many children who fail to respond to one type of stimulant medication respond very well to another stimulant.

Finally, don't make the mistake of thinking that with medication, less is always better than more. Parents who assume this stance often avoid giving medication late in the day and on weekends, even if the child has significant problems without medication. As Dr. Eist points out, "If your child has ADHD, he has it all day, every day." If he needs medication all day, every day, you do him a disservice by withholding medication afternoons and weekends.

Follow-up Care. Common sense dictates that youngsters should not simply be put on stimulant medication without professional oversight at regular intervals. However, several studies have documented that most children receive inadequate follow-up care. As children grow and change, their need for medication changes too. Sometimes an adjustment in dose or timing is all that is needed: the child's schedule changes when he enters middle school, for example, so the timing of medication must be adjusted accordingly.

In other cases, a medication that was once effective may no longer seem helpful. Sometimes an adjustment in dose is needed: although stimulants are no longer prescribed in doses that correspond to body weight, some children need slightly higher doses as they grow. Then there are children who seem to develop tolerance to medication over time, such that higher doses work only briefly, if at all, to control symptoms. True tolerance to the effects of stimulant medication is rare, however,[99] and often what appears to be tolerance is actually a response to some stress or crisis in the child's environment or to the emergence of another disorder, such as a mood disorder.

"Gary was diagnosed with ADHD when he was in kindergarten," his mother explained. "Ritalin helped him settle down and focus on his work. He had some problems midway through first grade—seemed kind of sourpuss and unhappy for a while—but that passed and he got back on track.

"He did fine in second grade, too, but this year has been bad news. His teacher says he can't follow directions and he never finishes his work. He's been having a lot of trouble getting along with the other kids too. We've tried increasing his Ritalin, but all that did was make him seem drugged."

When Gary's parents sought help from a child psychiatrist skilled in the use of medication, they were surprised to learn that Gary was depressed. An antidepressant was prescribed and, within a few weeks, Gary seemed like himself again. He still had some run-ins with two boys in his class who had targeted him for vicious teasing, but he and his therapist worked on ways to help him handle their attacks and to stand up for himself without bursting into tears.

If your child is doing well on medication, how often should you meet with the mental health professional who oversees your child's care? Dr. Eist recommends that appointments be scheduled monthly because, he points out, stressors can crop up and need for medication can change quickly. Regular follow-up visits are a good way to head off any emerging problems and to maintain contact with the professional in case you need services in a hurry at any point.

By the way, your child will be relieved to know that routine blood tests are *not* necessary as part of the monitoring process for Dexedrine, Adderal, or Ritalin.[100]

Adjunctive Interventions: When Are They Necessary?

What percentage of ADHD children respond well to stimulant medication? Of these, how many are then able to function in a manner comparable to that of their non-ADHD peers? These are tough questions to answer because most of the available information is based on children studied in research investigations—children who, as we have already discussed, tend to have more serious symptoms and more coexisting problems than ADHD children in the general population.

In general, however, if we combine research data and experience from clinical practice, it's safe to say that at least ninety percent of ADHD children are helped by stimulants. Of this group, some will show dramatic improvement across a variety of settings—so dramatic that no further intervention is needed. Others, however, will show improvement but continue to struggle at home or in school or both.

Obviously, these children need adjunctive interventions such as psychotherapy, behavior management programs, and/or educational remediation. In fact, experts now routinely cite the need for "multimodal treatment" for ADHD children and a five-year multisite investigation sponsored by the National Institute of Mental Health is now under way to study the questions of which ADHD children are likely to benefit from particular treatments and combinations of treatments.[101]

But the pendulum may have swung a bit too far. While there can be no doubt that many ADHD children do need other interventions in addition to medication, it's unsettling to hear a professional flatly state that "medication alone is never enough." This is simply not true, and it is confusing to parents of those ADHD youngsters for whom treatment with medication is quite sufficient.

Myths About Stimulants

Myths about stimulants have flourished like weeds, and, like weeds, they are very hard to kill. Among the most recurrent of these myths are the following:

- **Stimulants are addictive.** Stimulants do not result in addiction in ADHD children. On the contrary; some children resist taking stimulant medication because they do not like the way the medication makes them feel and people don't become addicted to substances that make them feel bad when they take them.

There is also no evidence that the use of stimulant medication predisposes youngsters to abuse illegal drugs.

Finally, it is fallacious to compare stimulants with drugs like cocaine: While there are pharmacological similarities between the two, there are important differences which make addiction to stimulants unlikely.[102]

- **Stimulants stunt growth.** Some reports in the 1970s suggested that long-term use of stimulant medication might stunt children's growth. Due to this concern, parents were urged to give children "drug holidays": a recommendation that was problematic for youngsters who simply couldn't function well without medication. More recent research[103] suggests that any height deficit in ADHD children reflects a temporarily slower growth tempo associated with ADHD itself rather than an effect of medication.

- **Stimulants can cause depression.** While some ADHD youngsters treated with stimulants develop depression, there is no evidence that stimulant treatment itself leads to depression. Instead, it appears likely that many ADHD children develop mood disorders completely independent of treatment with stimulant medication.
- **Stimulants don't work with adolescents.** In the past, it was thought that children outgrew their symptoms in adolescence and that stimulant medication would be of little or no help to youngsters whose problems continued into the teen years. We now know that people with ADHD continue to benefit from stimulant medication through adolescence and in the adult years as well.[104]

Recently, there have been reports of teenagers obtaining Ritalin from youngsters for whom it has been legitimately prescribed, grinding it into powder, and "snorting" it for a drug-induced high. But some misguided youngsters inhale the fumes from glue and other toxic substances to produce a high. Does this mean that we should ban these substances? I for one don't think so.

There has also been controversy about stimulants in ADHD individuals with tic disorders, particularly those with Tourette's syndrome (see Chapter 2). The evidence indicates that stimulants do not cause Tourette's syndrome (although they may "uncover" it in some cases) and that stimulants are generally a safe, effective treatment for the majority of ADHD children with tic disorder.[105] In fact, even when tics are slightly worsened by stimulant medication, some ADHD children and their parents elect to continue stimulant treatment if the cost-benefit ratio suggests that this is the best course of action. Treatment *must* be individualized for every child, however, and children with tics must be closely monitored on stimulant medication, since a few do have a worsening of tics on stimulants.[106]

When Stimulants Don't Work

There are ADHD children for whom stimulant medication is not helpful, at least when it is used alone and not as part of a combined medication regimen. Researchers estimate, for example, that as many as half to two-thirds of ADHD children with coexisting mood or anxiety disorders show little improvement in behavior, memory, or attention on stimulants alone. Some—perhaps as many as twenty-five percent—actually worsen in behavior on stimulants alone,[107,108] although many of these youngsters respond well to stimulants when their coexisting problems are treated with other medications.

When it comes to medication for your child, you *must* be watchful and observant. Regardless of how pleased others might be with your child's response to medication, if you don't like what you see—if your child seems to have lost his "spark," for example—consult your doctor about alternatives. Stimulant medication should enhance your child's ability to focus and control himself: it should never be used as a chemical strait-jacket.

Antidepressants

Tricyclic Antidepressants

Almost forty years ago, tricyclic antidepressants were found to be helpful in treating bedwetting. Not long afterward, reports appeared regarding their beneficial effects on symptoms of ADHD as well. To date, thirty or so studies have been conducted with over one thousand ADHD children and adults. The tricyclics imipramine (Tofranil) and desipramine (Norpramin) have been the most extensively studied, with more recent studies directed at desipramine, since it is less likely than imipramine to produce drowsiness, constipation, dry mouth, or impairments in fine motor control and memory.

In general, research has supported tricyclics as a good second-line medication for ADHD individuals who do not respond well to stimulants, leading to improvements in hyperactivity and aggression.[109] The effects of the tricyclics are longer-lasting than those of the stimulants, so there is better control of symptoms during the late afternoon and evening, without the complication of stimulant-induced insomnia. They also appear to have a weak but positive effect on mood and anxiety, neither of which is helped by stimulant medication. Since they do not usually cause a worsening of tics in ADHD youngsters who have Tourette's syndrome, the tricyclics are often used to treat ADHD symptoms in these patients. There is general agreement, however, that tricyclics are not as useful as stimulants, especially as concerns their effects on attention.

Tricyclics seem to be effective in a daily dose range of 1 to 5 milligrams for each kilogram of body weight. Some children do respond to fairly low doses, but improvement is not always sustained over time and increases in dose may be necessary.

Before these medications or any medication other than stimulants are prescribed, the child should have a physical examination and lab studies, including blood work and a urinalysis, as well as an electrocardiogram (EKG). Because the tricyclics can affect the electrical activity of the heart, heart rate and blood pressure should be monitored and repeat EKGs should be obtained as the dose of medication is increased. Thereafter, an EKG should be obtained annually—earlier, if the doctor finds the child's pulse abnormal. Tricyclics should never be stopped abruptly: to do so can result in flulike symptoms of nausea, stomach pain, vomiting, and headaches. Finally, like all other medications, the tricyclics should be kept securely beyond the reach of small children, because an overdose can be fatal.

The SSRIs: Prozac and Related Medications

When Prozac burst upon the scene in the 1980s, it marked the arrival of an entirely new class of antidepressants known as "SSRIs" (selective serotonin reuptake inhibitors). Prozac (fluoxetine) and its sister medicines, Zoloft (sertraline) and Paxil (paroxetine), are free of the annoying side effects that led many depressed patients to discontinue treatment with tricyclics in the past, and there can be no doubt that for many, these are truly life-saving medications.

The SSRIs heralded a new age in the treatment of both depression and obsessive compulsive disorder, but how effective are they in treating ADHD? Since the SSRIs act on the neurotransmitter serotonin, and since ADHD is more closely associated with problems in the dopamine system, it's not surprising that the track record of SSRIs with uncomplicated ADHD is fairly lackluster.

However, many child psychiatrists—both clinicians and researchers[110]—have also found that a combination of an SSRI and a stimulant can be extremely helpful with the ADHD child who has a coexisting mood disorder or an oppositional defiant disorder. In my own practice, I have seen a lot of angry, irritable children respond to an SSRI with improvement in mood and attitude: typical comments are "Things don't bug me as much now as they used to" and "I don't feel as mean and grouchy now." When a stimulant is then added to the regimen, these children report improvements in their ability to focus, organize themselves, and tackle their schoolwork.

Since research and clinical experience indicate that a starting dose of 20 mg. of Prozac can sometimes produce undesirable side effects (such as nausea, jitteriness, and increased anxiety), experienced clinicians usually begin with a smaller dose and build up to larger doses only gradually. The SSRIs certainly seem to be safe medications: they do not, for example, have the same cardiac side effects as the tricyclics, so there is no need for repeated EKGs. They are also much safer than the tricyclics if accidentally or deliberately taken in overdose: patients have survived after having taken amounts equal to at least ten times the daily dose.[111]

Wellbutrin

Wellbutrin (buproprion) is an antidepressant that doesn't fit into any other class of antidepressants. Because it seems to affect both dopamine and norepinephrine, it has been investigated as an alternative to stimulant medication in treating ADHD.

Research findings indicate that Wellbutrin is helpful with many of the symptoms of ADHD, although the stimulants are more effective, particularly as concerns effects on attention and concentration.[112,113] Studies of Wellbutrin with ADHD individuals have been short-term and there are some indications that the initial beneficial effects of Wellbutrin might not last more than a few weeks or months at best. Side effects experienced by some patients include skin rashes[114] and, more commonly, nausea. At higher doses, Wellbutrin should be carefully monitored in patients who have a history of seizures or eating disorders such as bulimia.

Effexor

Effexor (venlafaxine) is another antidepressant that doesn't fit into any other class of antidepressants. It works by affecting serotonin but, unlike the SSRIs, it also affects the neurotransmitters norepinephrine and, to a lesser extent, dopamine. Both of these neurotransmitters play a role in ADHD. There are early reports of success in treating ADHD adults with Effexor from at least three separate research groups.[115,116,117] Although Effexor seems particularly helpful for ADHD adults with coexisting mood or anxiety problems, very good effects—equal to those obtained with stimulants or with Wellbutrin—were also reported in those without such coexisting problems.

Unfortunately, Effexor often results in side effects of sedation, confusion, and nausea. In addition, a study of Effexor with ADHD children, most of whom had coexisting mood, anxiety, or conduct disorders, Effexor was helpful for some patients but actually worsened symptoms of hyperactivity in others.[118]

Other Medications

Clonidine

Catapres (clonidine), a blood pressure medication, reduces aggressive behavior, poor frustration tolerance, and noncompliant behavior in children who are severely overactive, aggressive, or explosive.[119] Clonidine is often particularly helpful in treating children who have both ADHD and a tic disorder: in these individuals, clonidine improves tic symptoms as well as impulsivity and restlessness and, in one study, improvement increased progressively across the twelve weeks of the study.[120]

Since clonidine does not improve distractibility, a combination of clonidine and Ritalin may be used to treat children who are highly aroused and distractible. Dr. Robert Hunt, the Vanderbilt University psychiatrist who pioneered explorations of clonidine with ADHD individuals, found that by combining the two medications, he could reduce doses of Ritalin by as much as forty percent in some individuals.[121]

Clonidine is usually administered three to four times daily, with meals and at bedtime. A skin patch that lasts for about five days eliminates the nuisance of multiple doses, but many children develop redness and itching at the site of the patch. There is also the danger that a young ADHD child (or a younger sibling) might suck or chew on the patch, thereby obtaining a lethal dose of the medication.

The most common side effect of clonidine is drowsiness, which is usually short-lived and can actually be beneficial when a bedtime dose is given to children with preexisting or medication-related sleep problems. Given clonidine before bed, the time it takes them to fall asleep is shortened considerably. A few have mild morning sedation, but this is usually not a problem: in fact, parents frequently report improvement in ADHD symptoms during the day, improvement that may be due to getting enough sleep.[122]

At the start of treatment, some children become slightly more irritable and moody, a side effect that can be minimized by increasing medication slowly. Depression has been reported in a small number of children, notably those who have a history or a family history of depression. Some children treated with clonidine at bedtime also report nightmares, which may be due to a rebound effect after about four or five hours.[123] These children would probably do better on guanfacine (brand name Tenex; see below). Children have been treated with clonidine for as long as five years without developing long-term side effects.[124]

Before clonidine is prescribed, the child should have a physical examination, blood studies and urinalysis, and an EKG, as is the case with all the medications discussed except the stimulants. The prescribing physician must also obtain a complete medical history, since clonidine may cause serious problems in children with preexisting heart disease or kidney problems. Children who take clonidine should have blood pressure and pulse checks weekly during the initial phase of treatment and at four- to six-week intervals after that. If the child takes clonidine during the day, it's very important that each dose be given on time and that no doses be skipped. And, like the tricyclics, clonidine should *never* be stopped abruptly. Instead, it should be gradually withdrawn under close supervision of a physician.

Guanfacine

Because the initial side effects of irritability and drowsiness are problems for some children treated with clonidine, Tenex (guanfacine) has recently been studied as an alternative. Guanfacine also has the advantage of a longer course of action, compared with clonidine.

Results of preliminary research with ADHD children appear promising: in studies with ADHD children, some of whom also had comorbid Tourette's syndrome, guanfacine produced improvements in attention, hyperactivity, impulsivity, aggression, frustration tolerance and—in those with Tourette's syndrome—in tics as well.[125,126] Not all children benefit from the medication, but in those who do, results are quite good and side effects are minimal. As is the case with clonidine, some children treated with guanfacine need lower doses of stimulants than when stimulants alone are used to treat ADHD.

Combinations of Medications: The New Trend

Just as mental health professionals have abandoned earlier attempts to identify a single overarching diagnosis for patients with multiple symptoms, psychiatrists are turning away from the search for a "magic bullet"—a single medication that would be effective in treating a broad array of symptoms such as we often see in ADHD children with coexisting conditions. Instead, there is a marked trend toward using two or more medications in combination to target specific symptoms.[127]

Combinations of medication are particularly likely to be used if there are two or more disorders present (e.g., a combination of an antidepressant and a stimulant to treat an ADHD youngster suffering from depression). A combination might also be prescribed if troublesome symptoms respond only partially to a single medication or if the physician thinks that two medicines, used together, will enable lower doses of each to be prescribed, thereby reducing side effects.

Medication regimens that involve two or more medications—especially if one is a newer medication such as Prozac—are often frightening to parents, many of whom are uneasy even with the use of even a single, well-studied medication such as Ritalin or Dexedrine. As a scientist, I wish I could report that we have data from long-term, controlled investigations concerning the use of these medications and these combinations in children. As a clinician, however, I have seen how helpful such medications and combinations of medication can be when prescribed by a professional skilled in psychopharmacology.

Sometimes parents ask me point blank, "What would you do if it were your child?" Since I work with extremely knowledgeable and experienced child psychiatrists, I am able to answer honestly that I would follow their recommendations, at least for a trial period. However, I would want to know:

- How long a trial period is anticipated?
- What specific benefits might result?
- What side effects might we see?
- What is the fallback plan if this approach doesn't work?

I might also want to get a second opinion, something parents often shy away from because they believe it is insulting to the professional involved. I don't see it that way: when my patients ask for a second opinion, I am grateful to have the benefit of another professional's expertise, particularly in more complicated cases, and I am more than happy to collaborate.

The Decision to Use Medication

Contrary to what some critics claim, most parents of ADHD children do not turn to medication because they are seeking an easy way out. In spite of all of the evidence—over 150 controlled studies and years and years of clinical experience—indicating that stimulants are the most effective treatment for ADHD, many parents are understandably reluctant to undertake a trial of medication for their child's problems.

With such parents, I would never argue or insist: instead, I agree to work with the family using alternative interventions, such as behavior therapy programs at home and in school. I do insist, however, that parents keep careful records of progress so that we can track the effectiveness of what we do. When, after six months to a few years, these parents ultimately decide to pursue treatment with medication, they can do so knowing that they have exhausted all other reasonable remedies.

The Child's Concerns

When a diagnosis of ADHD is presented in a way that children can understand it, most youngsters are at least moderately receptive to taking medication to help with their difficulties. Some, in fact, are quite enthusiastic. Others, however—especially teenagers—resist the idea, sometimes to the point of outright refusal. What can we do in such a situation?

It depends on the situation. When the parent of a six-year-old asks, "What if he won't take the medicine?" I know that a lot of work needs to be done on other issues besides medication—issues of oppositional and defiant behavior—since it is not up to a six-year-old to decide whether or not he will take medication prescribed for him.

Some children who object to medication have legitimate concerns. Some, mindful of the dangers of drug abuse, worry that they might become addicted. Others fear being teased and humiliated by their peers and stigmatized as "weird" or "crazy." As a parent, you can help allay these fears by simply hearing the child out, without arguing or debating. When you are sure that you understand your child's objections, try to solve the problem with him: "Let's put our heads together and see if we can come up with some good solutions to the problem."

With adolescents, however, the situation can be much stickier. Adolescents are involved in the process of moving away from the control of others toward their own autonomy. It's an anxious time, a time when fitting in with the all-important peer group assumes paramount significance. At such a time, it's no wonder that some adolescents adamantly reject a diagnosis and a treatment that sets them apart from their peers or that challenges their autonomy. Young people in this age group are particularly apt to insist "I can do it myself. I don't need a pill to help me." Some fear that taking medication would prove they are crazy or that the medication might damage their body or change their personality.

One tactic that may be helpful with resistant adolescents is to provide them with books and articles about ADHD and the medications used to treat it.* In fact, researchers have found that providing teens with written information about their psychiatric condition and their medication leads to increased knowledge and to an improvement in attitude toward taking psychotropic medication.[128]

But what about the teenager who adamantly refuses to undertake a trial of medication or who decides to discontinue medication in spite of evidence that the medication is helpful to him? In my experience, such youngsters often return to treatment when the ability to concentrate and pay attention becomes important to them—when, for example, poor grades threaten their eligibility to play on a school athletic team or to get into the college of their choice.

In the meantime, you as a parent must realize that you cannot force-feed medication to an adolescent unless life-threatening circumstances are involved. (Note: Flunking algebra is not usually considered life-threatening!) Painful as it might be for you, you will probably just have to give in with as much grace as you can muster. Instead of an all-or-nothing situation, however, try to negotiate a compromise: for example, if the teenager agrees to have his assignment sheet initialed by his teachers every day and to attend tutoring, the question of medication will be deferred.

---

* One youngster was willing to read my book, *Distant Drums, Different Drummers,* and even write a brief review of the book, when his savvy mother told him he would be paid for his efforts.

CHAPTER 6

WHAT ELSE CAN WE DO? PSYCHOTHERAPY AND TRAINING APPROACHES

Overview: Then and Now

Then: A decade ago, most professionals urged parents to explore all other avenues of intervention before turning to medication. Behavior therapy techniques were touted as particularly helpful for ADHD children. Many professionals also hoped that ADHD youngsters might benefit from cognitive therapy to help them think before acting, although results of research even at that time were discouraging.

Now: Medication is now recognized by most experts as a first line of treatment for ADHD, although there is agreement that many ADHD children and adolescents also need adjunctive treatment such as behavior therapy or some other form of psychotherapy. The role of psychotherapy in the treatment of ADHD has been much more clearly defined: while core symptoms of ADHD do not respond to treatment with psychotherapy, many ADHD individuals with coexisting psychiatric problems can benefit from psychotherapy. In order to obtain the best treatment for their children, parents need to be knowledgeable about the various forms of psychotherapy available.

What Is Psychotherapy?

Eight-year-old Meg was generally an agreeable youngster. Let something go wrong, however—a disagreement with a friend, a teasing remark from her older brother—and Meg fell apart, wailing that nobody loved her and that she wanted to die. After her dog died, she developed sleep and appetite problems and became increasingly withdrawn and irritable. When this behavior persisted for several weeks, her parents sought professional help.

At first, Meg was restrained with Dr. Sanders and noncommittal when her parents asked how her visits went. Soon, however, she began to look forward to the sessions, in which she and Dr. Sanders talked, drew pictures, made figures from modeling clay, and played games that involved talking about feelings of fear, anger, and sadness.

When, after several sessions, Meg's mother reported improved sleep and appetite, Meg nodded enthusiastically and agreed, "Yeah, that's really true." In subsequent sessions, Dr. Sanders helped Meg acknowledge and confront some half-buried fears about harm befalling her parents or herself through some negligent act on her part. Meg's mother or father sat in for at least a few minutes during most sessions, getting feedback from Dr. Sanders and providing information about Meg's day-to-day functioning.

At the end of a year, Dr. Sanders, Meg, and Meg's parents agreed that Meg was doing so well that she no longer needed regular visits with Dr. Sanders. Visits were tapered to monthly, and after three months, therapy was terminated with the understanding that Meg's parents would call Dr. Sanders if problems cropped up in the future.

Sometimes called "the talking cure," the term psychotherapy encompasses a wide variety of methods and techniques aimed at helping people make changes in their attitudes, emotions, and behavior patterns. The goals of psychotherapy can range from the narrowly circumscribed—for example, helping a person who suffers from intense fear of flying learn to tolerate air travel—to the very broad and global, such as helping a patient develop more satisfying relationships with family, friends, coworkers, and employers.

The methods, too, and the assumptions about human behavior on which they are based, vary enormously. For example, following in the footsteps of Sigmund Freud, *psychodynamic therapists* seek to help patients recognize and come to grips with the unconscious conflicts, fears, and fantasies that interfere with their ability to cope with the demands of everyday life.

In contrast, *behavior therapists* do not assume that disturbed behavior stems from underlying unconscious conflict. Instead, they believe that specific behaviors are learned because they produce specific consequences which the individual experiences as either positive or negative. By altering the consequences that follow behavior, behavior therapists aim to alter behavior directly, thereby improving the way in which the individual functions.

Cognitive therapists take a similarly direct approach to treating disturbed behavior. By teaching people to identify, challenge, and change patterns of self-defeating thought, beliefs, and attitudes, cognitive therapists seek to bring about changes in emotions and behavior. Cognitive therapy techniques have been applied to a variety of problems, including those characteristic of ADHD as well as symptoms of depression and anxiety disorders.

As we shall see, *family therapy* can take many forms. Sometimes the term family therapy is used to refer generally to any type of therapy in which other family members, including parents, are directly involved. Sometimes, however, the term refers to a specific way of thinking about how children's disturbed behavior reflects disturbances in the overall functioning in the family.

Group therapy, too, can take several forms. In group therapy, the child is helped to see what effects his behavior has on others and how his own behavior causes problems for him. The group serves as a safe place in which the child can work on these problems and try out new, more satisfying ways of behaving. Group therapy can be insight-oriented or the group can be used as the setting in which specific skills are taught directly, such as social-skills groups.

While these approaches seem very different from each other, in actual practice they have much in common. In practice, too, therapists trained in one "school" often borrow methods and techniques from other schools to help them treat the problems their patients experience. Dr.

Norman Rosenthal, a skilled clinician and a well-known scientist, put it beautifully when he described himself as "quite suspicious of people who believe that only one narrow school of thought carries the key to curing all psychological problems." "People," he added, "are far too diverse and complicated for such simple solutions."[129]

Is psychotherapy effective? This question has been hotly debated by behavioral scientists at least since the early 1950s, when the first outcome studies of psychotherapy were undertaken, and several entire books have been written on the subject. Certainly, there are numerous studies, including the recent large-scale survey conducted by *Consumer Reports*,[130] indicating that people who undergo psychotherapy of one form or another benefit from it. The question itself, however, is too broad to be answered with a simple yes or no. Instead of asking whether "psychotherapy works," we should ask what specific forms of therapy and which specific procedures are most effective in dealing with specific clinical problems.

You cannot be an informed consumer unless you understand the different forms of therapy available to you, your ADHD child, and your family. To help you understand how these various forms of therapy may be of help to your child, let's examine each in a bit more detail.

Psychodynamic Psychotherapy

Because this form of psychotherapy focuses on helping people gain understanding and insight into their unconscious conflicts, it is often referred to as insight-oriented psychotherapy. Therapists who work in this fashion use a variety of techniques, including free association (saying anything that comes into one's mind) and dream analysis to uncover and explore material buried in the unconscious mind—material that the patient has repressed because it is too awful to think about consciously.

Insight-oriented therapists who work with children use puppets, dolls, art materials, games, and toys to help them understand the child's fears, needs, and inner turmoil. Through play, the child's natural "language," the child is helped to work through and master the painful and frightening material buried in his unconscious. As this material is gradually brought to light and the child sees that neither he nor the therapist suffers a horrible fate as a result, the child begins to come to grips with painful memories and frightening thoughts. As he does, his inner distress subsides and he is able to behave and interact with others in a more appropriate and satisfying manner.

The Bottom Line

Does psychodynamic psychotherapy work for ADHD children? Since the core problems associated with ADHD—impulsivity, hyperactivity, and attentional difficulties—are caused by differences in the way the ADHD child's brain functions, it is not surprising that these problems do not respond to a treatment approach aimed at resolving underlying *emotional* problems. On the other hand, for the emotional problems such as anxiety, depression, and poor self-esteem that often coexist with ADHD, it is the general consensus among experts that psychodynamic psychotherapy can be of considerable benefit.[131]

What are the drawbacks? Since the goal of psychodynamic psychotherapy is to unearth material buried in the unconscious, this form of therapy can be rather lengthy, sometimes going on for a couple of years. Some insight-oriented psychotherapists do work adjunctively with parents, but, for the most part, the emphasis is on working directly with the child and parents sometimes complain that they are pretty much in the dark concerning what is going on with their child's therapy.

Cognitive Therapy

The approach to changing behavior and emotions that is known as cognitive therapy was developed along different lines by mental health professionals who worked with patients with different types of problems.

Cognitive Training for ADHD

In Canada, Dr. Virginia Douglas, a psychologist widely known for her research in the area of ADHD, thought that the primary problem of the

ADHD child was his inability to "stop, look and listen." Following her lead, psychologists developed a number of cognitive training programs designed to teach ADHD children to think their way through problems and tasks by applying a prescribed series of questions and rules to their own behavior. For example, when confronting an academic task, the ADHD child was taught to ask himself, "What is the problem?" and "What is it I have to do?" The child was taught to check his progress at each step along the way and to review his work for careless errors.

After initial training on tasks such as puzzles and mazes, ADHD children were taught to apply their new skills to schoolwork and to social situations. For example, programs were designed to help ADHD children cope with difficult peer situations in a less impulsive fashion, with training that included social problem-solving skills, role playing, and exercises to teach cooperation with others.

Researchers then tested these programs, but with disappointing results. Under the direction of skilled researchers, programs were undertaken in Chicago at the University of Illinois and in New York at Columbia University.[132,133] At the conclusion of these very well-designed programs, researchers found that cognitive training did not reduce the need for stimulant medication, nor did it result in improved classroom behavior, academic gains, or improvement in social behavior. In short, cognitive therapy for ADHD proved to be something of a bust!

Cognitive Therapy for Other Psychiatric Conditions

At about the same time psychologists were exploring the use of cognitive treatment for ADHD, other mental health professionals were applying cognitive therapy to different kinds of problems. At the University of Pennsylvania, psychiatrist Dr. Aaron Beck observed that depressed people have maladaptive ways of thinking about themselves, the world, and the future. These disturbed ways of thinking, he came to believe, contributed to maladaptive ways of behaving.

Specifically, Dr. Beck found that depressed people see themselves as defective, inept, and inadequate and that when bad things happen to them, they take it as proof that they are worthless and deserving of ill fortune. Depressed people also have a negative view of their world, interpreting everything that happens in the worst possible light. Finally, since depressed people believe they are fundamentally flawed, they assume that their problems will continue—that the future will be at least as bleak as the present, if not more so.

Dr. Beck then developed techniques to help depressed people identify, challenge, and change these maladaptive ways of thinking. For example, a youngster who gets a bad grade on a test might be taught to challenge resulting thoughts of "I'm stupid. Nothing I do ever works out" and to replace them with more rational and less self-defeating thoughts, such as "I've done pretty well on other tests. I'll have to study harder the next time."

In practice, the methods developed by Dr. Beck are usually combined with methods devised by Dr. Albert Ellis,[134] another pioneer in cognitive therapy. Dr. Ellis developed the "ABC model," which explains how what we believe (B) about an adverse event (A) results in how we feel as a consequence (C). If, for example, a friend lets me down and I tell myself "How awful after all I've done for her—she should have been there for me!" I'm setting myself up to feel furious. On the other hand, if I tell myself, "I'm disappointed in her, but nobody's perfect." I'll at least stay calm enough to talk over the problem with my friend and I won't make myself miserable with rage in the meantime. As Dr. Ellis would point out, it's not the event itself (my friend's behavior) that causes me to feel angry; it's what I tell myself about the event that determines how I feel and how I behave as a result.

Cognitive therapy has been used with both children and adults who suffer from depression. In addition, mental health professionals have expanded the use of these techniques to the treatment of individuals who suffer from various forms of anxiety disorders.

The Bottom Line

Cognitive therapy, applied to the core symptoms of ADHD, appears to have little or nothing to offer as a primary means of intervention. This finding is particularly disappointing to parents, for whom cognitive therapy has particular appeal since it seemed to offer the hope that ADHD children could learn strategies for controlling their own behavior, thereby eventually eliminating the need for medication.

On the other hand, cognitive therapy does appear to hold considerable promise for helping youngsters who have coexisting mood and anxiety disorders. Cognitive therapy has been shown to benefit children with these problems and that children maintain the gains they make in therapy.[135]

Parents can—and should—be actively involved in their youngster's program of cognitive therapy so that they can provide appropriate support and coaching in applying the techniques in daily life. A good resource is *The Optimistic Child,* written by Dr. Martin Seligman.* Dr. Seligman is a pioneer in the application of cognitive therapy with depressed children and adolescents and his own research has demonstrated the benefits of this type of therapy.

Family Therapy

The term "family therapy" is particularly confusing for parents, who assume that it refers simply to therapy in which parents are actively involved in the child's ongoing treatment. The term appeals to parents of ADHD children because many are acutely aware of the difficulties their ADHD child's behavior causes in the family. Many, too, long to develop a more satisfying, effective, and less punitive way of relating to their ADHD children.

In reality, however, family therapy can mean different things to different people. Therapists from vastly different backgrounds may include family members in therapy sessions as part of the child's ongoing psychotherapy. In contrast, mental health professionals who have been specifically trained in "strategic family therapy" or "structural family therapy" view the *family,* not the *child,* as the patient because they assume that the child's problems result from disturbances in the way the family operates as a system. For example, there may be marital difficulties that make the child feel insecure and vulnerable, or a parent may suffer from depression or some other psychiatric disorder. Some family therapists see the child's symptoms as serving some covert purpose in the system, such as distract-

* Boston: Houghton Mifflin, 1995.

ing feuding parents from their battles, thereby holding their marriage together.

It is the job of the family therapist to identify and correct the underlying systemic problems by improving communication in the family, teaching problem-solving skills, and helping parents reestablish their position as authority figures. When this is accomplished, it is assumed that the child's problems will clear up without additional intervention.

The Bottom Line

As is the case with other types of psychotherapy, family therapy does not alter the core symptoms of ADHD. However, family therapy may be useful in identifying misunderstandings among family members and in helping parents work together to manage an ADHD child more effectively. In addition, joint sessions with parents and children can provide a forum in which the concerns of all can be addressed and compromises negotiated.

Turning to research, studies have shown that family therapy can help improve child behavior and family interaction in at least some families.[136] Surprisingly, this approach seems particularly effective with conduct-disordered adolescents, a group notoriously refractory to other types of treatment.[137]

Parents considering this type of therapy should be forewarned, however: because the child's problems are seen as resulting from family problems, it is not uncommon for family therapists to dismiss children from the sessions after just a few appointments to focus on marital problems or other adult issues.[138] In addition, many family therapists have little training in working with children and so tend to avoid it if possible. This means that the problems for which you sought treatment in the first place might not be the focus of treatment. It also means that coexisting problems in the ADHD child are likely to be overlooked.

Group Therapy

Strictly speaking, group therapy is not a specific type of therapy: rather, many types of therapy can be offered in a group setting, as opposed to individual work.

Twenty years ago, while on the faculty at the West Virginia University Medical School, I hit upon what I thought was the brilliant idea of putting ADHD children (then called "hyperactive") into groups for therapy. Russell Barkley happened to be visiting WVU around that time to give a talk about his research and, when I eagerly described my plan, he commented, "How interesting. I don't know of anyone else who is doing that."

I soon found out why! I had only a vague notion of what I hoped to accomplish in the group and how to go about it. Without a well-thought-out plan, my group of bouncy, active, impulsive youngsters—several of whom were not on medication—quickly spiraled out of control. Very soon thereafter, the group was disbanded, much to the relief of my colleagues and students who were involved in the project.

Today, therapists are much more sophisticated and savvy. Working with small groups of ADHD children whose impulsivity and hyperactivity are minimized by medication, they help ADHD children who are socially isolated or who think that ADHD means that they are weird, different, or defective come to terms with ADHD. The school setting is the most logical place in which to offer such groups, which are usually organized and led by the school guidance counselor following teacher referral and parent permission for the child to participate. In my experience, children who have participated in such "friendship groups" have found them to be enormously helpful. To my great delight, in fact, one youngster who had enjoyed participating in such a group wrote a note to her counselor the following year, urging that the group be reconvened in the new academic year.

The Bottom Line

In settings outside of the school, specialized groups for ADHD children are often very difficult to find. This is unfortunate, because meeting other children with similar problems can be so beneficial to ADHD youngsters. Talking about common concerns often forms the basis for friendships among the children and receiving acceptance and support from others who are in the same boat can be very gratifying to children with ADHD.

If you think your child might benefit from such a group but you are unable to locate one, ask the guidance counselor at your child's school if he or she would consider starting such a group.

Behavior Therapy: Engineering the Environment

Behavior therapy, sometimes called "behavior modification," is the form of mental health intervention with which parents of ADHD children are most familiar, since this approach seems tailor made for many of the problems faced by ADHD children.

What It Is and How It Works

Behavior therapy involves arranging the environment so that pleasant, enjoyable things happen when the child (or animal) behaves appropriately and that these things are removed following inappropriate or undesirable behavior. Based largely on the work of Harvard psychologist B. F. Skinner, the overriding principle of behavior therapy is that behavior is affected most strongly by consequences that immediately follow the behavior. Thus, a puppy who is rewarded with a biscuit learns to come when he is called and a toddler learns to say "please" if this behavior results in a cookie. Similarly, we turn up the thermostat on chilly days because we have learned that this action produces the welcome sensation of warmth.

When there is no "payoff" for a behavior, the behavior tends to weaken and eventually stop altogether. You would not keep putting coins in a candy machine that did not reward your behavior with a candy bar, nor would you continue to wave at a neighbor who never returned your greeting. You would cease your efforts even more abruptly if, instead of an absence of positive consequences, you encountered unpleasant or painful consequences—if you received a shock from the vending machine, for example, or if your neighbor cursed at you in response to your greeting.

Consequences need not be dramatic in order to affect behavior: a smile can be a very effective positive consequence; a frown can serve as a negative consequence, bringing a particular behavior to a halt. Such social consequences can be surprisingly effective in strengthening or weakening behavior, because Mother Nature has designed us such that we yearn for and respond to praise and approval from others of our own species.

Social consequences—indeed, all consequences—provide us with essential information about our own behavior. Positive consequences tell us that our behavior is on the right track, just as route markers along the highway tell the motorist he is going in the right direction. Conversely, negative consequences signal an error and tell us to change direction. (An important point to note about negative consequences is that they tell us only what *doesn't* work: they don't provide information about what we should do instead.)

To emphasize the informational properties of positive consequences, I prefer to use the technical term "reinforcer" rather than "reward." Because "reward" implies a special treat for special effort, "rewarding" good behavior seems strange and artificial to many parents. Some see this as bribery; others worry that the approach will cost them a fortune.

The term "reinforcement" carries no such connotations, calls up no visions of daily trips to the toy store. "To reinforce" simply means "to strengthen" and the best way to strengthen a behavior is to follow it with positive consequences. Cast in this light, providing positive reinforcement for behavior makes very good sense.

Using Positive Consequences

Positive consequences, or reinforcers, are the most potent tool in a good behavior management program, and how you select and use them will determine the success of your program. You must, for example, use reinforcers that are meaningful to your child. As a parent, you are in the best position to know what your child most values and enjoys.

What Can You Use? Many of the everyday activities your child enjoys—watching television, talking on the telephone, playing computer games—can be incorporated into a behavior management program. To a great extent, successful use of these reinforcers depends on how you present them. For example, it's more effective to say "When you finish your homework, you may go out to play," instead of "You can't go out to play if you don't finish your homework."

Here are some other tips to keep in mind when selecting reinforcers:

▪ **Avoid the "goodies trap."** Instead of buying special treats, use items you would ordinarily purchase for the child and let him earn them. With expensive items, you can get maximum mileage with a "rental program"; that is, the child earns the privilege of using the item on a daily or weekly basis. For example, instead of promising the child a stereo if he makes good grades, buy the stereo and let him rent it on a weekly basis, based on satisfactory grades and homework for the week. This lets you provide your child with a coveted item without bankrupting you. It also avoids long delay between good behavior and the reinforcer, delays during which the ADHD child is apt to become discouraged and give up.

▪ **Use lots of praise.** Praise, attention, and approval are the most potent positive consequences in your armamentarium, believe it or not. Smiles, winks, and hugs don't cost a cent, but they yield huge dividends in good behavior.

If, like most of us, you tend to be too generous with criticism and too stingy with praise, try this little experiment. Divide an index card into columns marked "praise" and "criticism." For three days, check the appropriate column each time you praise or criticize your child for something he is doing. If you find that you're doling out a lot more criticism than praise, try this strategy: put ten pennies or beans in your pocket and transfer one to the other pocket every time you praise your child. To make it most effective, promise yourself that you won't say a critical word until you've transferred all ten markers from one pocket to the other.

You'll probably be surprised at how well this approach works. You may be surprised, too, to find that your other children take a turn for the better as well, since the beneficial effects of praise tend to spill over even to those who don't directly experience the praise. You'll feel better, too, since it's so much more fun to compliment good behavior than to punish bad behavior.

Remember, too, that overheard compliments are a potent way to deliver praise for good behavior. Let your child overhear you praising a specific example of his good behavior to your spouse or to a neighbor. Be specific—"Pat made her bed this morning and did a great job of putting all her toys away"—so the child knows exactly what behaviors met with your approval.

Using Positive Consequences: Points to Remember. Since reinforcers are used to signal "That's right; keep it up," they provide the most effective feedback when they follow hot on the heels of a desirable behavior. ADHD children, in particular, seek immediate reinforcement and are very susceptible to delays between behavior and reinforcement.

Other points to remember:

■ **Be generous; reinforce often.** Scientists who have observed the performance of ADHD children in the laboratory report that overall performance improves markedly when reinforcers are delivered frequently. When reinforcers are few and far between, the behavior of ADHD children deteriorates more rapidly than that of other children. Remember that reinforcers are behavioral "route markers" and use them frequently to help your ADHD child stay on the right road.

■ **Reinforce small steps toward improvement.** Probably the single most common mistake parents make in using behavior management programs is offering a huge payoff for a huge amount of improvement. Remember that ADHD children live very much in the present and have an I-want-it-now! approach to life. Promising such a youngster a deal like "If you don't fight with your sister for a month, I'll buy you a puppy" is futile, since the ADHD youngster has about as much chance of achieving this goal as he does of winning the lottery—maybe even less! Instead, offer small reinforcers for goals that are actually within the child's reach, such as an extra hour of computer time on days when no sibling altercations occur.

■ **Don't reinforce what hasn't yet happened.** Another common mistake is to reinforce a behavior before it occurs, instead of afterward.

PARENT: If I let you watch TV now, you have to promise that you'll do
   your homework this evening.

CHILD: Sure, I promise.

Notice that what is being reinforced here is *not* the desired behavior (doing homework) but the behavior of making a promise. Unfortunately, many ADHD children are quick to make promises but woefully slow in keeping them.

You can avoid this dilemma by keeping in mind a simple, old-fashioned rule: "Work before you play."

Using Negative Consequences

Parents are sometimes taken aback by the emphasis on positive consequences, because this focus is the reverse of our usual approach to discipline. When we think of discipline, we tend to think first of putting a stop to problem behavior, and punishment is the first method that comes to mind.

This is unfortunate, indeed, because punishment is generally an ineffective and inefficient way to improve behavior. There are several problems with punishment, as we shall see.

Problems with Punishment. Unlike positive consequences, punishing consequences only signal "Stop." They don't tell the child what he should do instead. Thus, if you spank your child for teasing the dog, for example, the child has to come up with another way to amuse himself. And, of course, with an ADHD child, the alternative activity of his choice is likely to be equally unacceptable—throwing rocks, say, or cutting holes in his bedspread.

While punishment can bring about an immediate halt to undesirable behavior, in the long run it often backfires and can actually lead to *in-*

creases in undesirable behavior. We know, for example, that children who are subjected to frequent spankings and other forms of physical punishment are particularly likely to behave aggressively toward their peers.

Punishment also has an adverse effect on the one who doles it out: parents of ADHD children often feel guilty about the fact that their interactions with their child are so negative in nature. Oftentimes, too, parents find themselves at odds over when and how to punish their children.

"Our home is like a war zone. It seems like all I do is scream at Lee. Every day I promise myself that we're going to make it through the day with no nagging or spanking. Then Lee does something like hit the neighbor kid or write on the bedroom walls and—bam!—there we go again!"

"My husband is constantly on Tracy's case. No wonder she says she's no good and that she can't do anything right. I tell him that he shouldn't be so hard on her, but if I step in we get into a fight about how we should handle her. That makes him furious, so he's twice as hard on her the next time. It's really gotten out of hand, but I don't know how to stop it."

Obviously, there are many problems associated with using punishment, especially with ADHD children. Does this mean you should rely exclusively on positive consequences to manage your child's behavior? Absolutely not! Such an approach is unrealistic and it wouldn't work even if you could manage to do it. Research shows that positive consequences alone are not enough: certain kinds of negative consequences are necessary, too, to keep behavior on the right track.

It does mean, however, that you should change the way you think about and use punishment. Begin by eliminating the term "punishment" from your vocabulary and even from your thinking. Replace it with "negative consequence" or "negative feedback." These terms remind you that your role in managing your child's behavior is that of a teacher or guide rather than a police officer or a warden.

Negative Consequences: What Can You Use? Negative consequences should not be harsh or painful. The point is to steer the child away from bad behavior, not to hurt or humiliate him, as traditional forms of punishment often do.

■ **Time-out.** The method known as "time-out," now widely used by parents, teachers, and others who work with children, is an outstanding example of a negative consequence that does not entail scolding, anger, or pain. This approach involves isolating the child for a few minutes after he misbehaves. Any boring place in the house will do nicely—a chair in the dining room, the stairs to the basement—just be sure it's quiet and isolated.

Don't think of time-out as a punishment. Instead, think of it as both a signal to the child that his behavior is unacceptable and as providing an opportunity for the child to cool off and pull himself together. With younger children, the mere act of removing them from an enjoyable activity for a few minutes can convey the message. With older children, time-out can be used to help them learn to leave the scene for a few minutes to cool off when they and/or the situation gets overheated. This is, in fact, a good lesson for children to practice for the future, particularly ADHD children, who tend to get "stuck" in a situation and escalate it into an explosion. Therefore, it's a good idea to specifically label time-out as an opportunity for the child to calm down and get his act together.

POOR: "You bad boy! Just for that, you have to go to time-out. Get in there right now!"

GOOD: "Hitting your brother is against the rules. Go into time-out for ten minutes and think about what you might have done instead."

Volumes of research have been written about how time-out should be utilized for greatest effect. Experts generally agree that time-out should be brief (one minute for each year of the child's age is a good rule of thumb); that the child must be quiet during the time-out or the clock will be reset; and that the time should be spent in a location away from television, toys, and other family members. Experts also agree that you should be calm and matter-of-fact when you send the child into time-out—no yelling, no lectures, no arguing or lengthy explanations and exhortations.

Time-out can also be used if your child misbehaves when you are away from home: use the car, a rest room, or a quiet corner as a time-out spot, or tell the child that he will have a time-out as soon as you return home.

Over the years, I've learned to expect lots of "What-if?" questions about time-out from parents of ADHD children. "What if my child refuses to go to time-out?" "What if he won't stay there?" "What if he trashes his room during time-out?" These behaviors are symptomatic not of ADHD, but of oppositional defiant disorder. I agree with the advice of Dr. Russell Barkley that parents should not undertake a behavior management program with a seriously oppositional/defiant child without professional help. Dr. Barkley has designed a special program to be implemented by mental health professionals working with these children.[139]

■ **Penalties** Penalties for unacceptable behavior usually consist of removing specific privileges, such as loss of the telephone or restriction to the house ("grounding"). If this doesn't work effectively with your child, you may have overlooked some of the finer points of this method. If, for example, you use long-term penalties or remove virtually all the child's privileges, the child may decide "I might as well do what I want: I've got nothing else to lose." Another problem with long-term penalties is that parents may find themselves trapped if they've grounded the child and a truly special occasion comes up. As a rule of thumb, a penalty should be in effect for no longer than a day, at most, for every five years of the child's age. Longer penalties are not more effective: they are just more difficult to enforce.

As an alternative to grounding a child or removing privileges, I prefer to impose penalties in the form of *community service,* especially if the child's behavior caused inconvenience or expense to another person. Work penalties, such as washing the car, cleaning the bathrooms, and weeding the garden do involve effort on your part because it's likely that you will have to supervise the child's work. However, this approach has the advantage of allowing the child to make restitution for misbehavior and wipe the slate clean.

When nine-year-old Alan arrived home an hour late for the second time in a week, his mother explained, "Since I spent almost an hour looking for you, you'll have to pay me back. I want you to weed the flower bed in front of the house. If you start right now, you should be finished in time for dinner."

Grumbling and sulking, Alan set about weeding the flower bed with little enthusiasm. His pace quickened considerably, however, after his mother appeared on the front porch and informed him pleasantly that she hoped he would finish in an hour so he wouldn't miss dinner. An hour later, the job completed to his mother's satisfaction, Alan sat down to dinner with his family.

How to Use Negative Consequences. If negative consequences don't seem to have much impact on your child's behavior, part of the problem may lie with the way you have been using them, as this example illustrates.

After a trying day, you have just collapsed on the couch with ten minutes all to yourself to read the paper. The kids are playing on the floor, Peter with his big trucks, Sarah with building blocks.

Out of the corner of your eye, you notice that Peter is moving his trucks with increasing force, occasionally bumping them into the walls and furniture. "Oh, no," you think, "I'm just too tired to handle any more trouble. Maybe if I just ignore it, he'll stop."

But Peter, being Peter, doesn't stop—he never does. With your last ounce of patience you say, "Peter, please stop being so rough with your trucks." No reply. The bumps become thumps. "Peter!" you warn in a louder tone. No reply. The thumps become crashes and the inevitable happens: Peter crashes a truck into his sister's block structure and his sister shrieks in protest.

You explode. "Dammit!" you yell, leaping up from the couch. "Can't you ever listen to me?" Grabbing him roughly by the arm, you jerk him toward the stairs. "Get upstairs and get ready for bed. I don't even want to have to look at you any more today."

Peter stomps up the stairs and into his room, slamming the door. You sink into a chair, angry and upset. "It never ends with that kid," you think. "It just never, never ends."

This little scenario illustrates several mistakes parents make in using negative consequences.

■ **Ignoring misbehavior usually doesn't work.** Parents are sometimes advised to ignore mild misbehavior on the assumption that the behavior will wither away if it is not reinforced with attention. Most parents find that this is difficult to do and, with ADHD children, usually ineffective, since ADHD children have problems putting the brakes on their own behavior. Parents, then, have to help by intervening actively when misbehavior occurs.

- **Don't nag.** Telling a child the same thing over and over is exasperating. When you want your child to stop what he is doing, don't give repeated warnings: tell him once, pleasantly but firmly, to stop, then be prepared to impose the consequences immediately.

- **Suggest and reinforce appropriate alternatives.** Because ADHD children find it so hard to inhibit their behavior, it is usually easier for them to stop doing something if they are redirected into another activity. For example, the parent in the example might have said, "Peter, no rough play in the living room. If you want to play with your trucks, please take them into your bedroom. If you stay in this room, you can watch television or you can color with your new crayons."

Redirecting is much more successful if it is accompanied by actual physical guidance.* Put your hand on the child's shoulder to gently propel him in the desired direction, for example, or help him pick up his toys to take them to another area.

- **Intervene early.** Don't wait until you are out of patience and your child is out of control before stepping in. The time to intervene is as early as possible. Although some parents object, "But I'd be on his back constantly if I stepped in for every little thing," intervening quickly to correct and redirect the child greatly reduces the number of times you will actually have to impose negative consequences.

A terrific variant of time-out known as "1-2-3 magic" lets you intervene quickly to nip problems in the bud without nagging or arguing. With this method, developed by psychologist Tom Phelan,[140] you calmly give a warning at the first sign of trouble by holding up one finger and saying, "That's one." If the behavior stops, fine, if not, you hold up two fingers and say, "That's two." If the behavior still doesn't stop within ten

---

* With some ADHD youngsters who tend to overfocus and become "stuck" in an activity, you must first gain the child's attention before you can redirect him. A good tactic with these children is to teach them, through lots of reinforced practice, to clasp their hands in front of them and make eye contact with you when you say "Listen up." When hands and eyes are thus removed from the ongoing activity, it is much easier to direct the child's attention to another activity.

seconds or so, you hold up three fingers and say, "That's three—take five" and send the child to his room for five minutes. Dr. Phelan cautions that in using this approach, you must remember to give an explanation only once and to refrain from saying anything else during the counting process.

Example

CHILD: Can I spend the night at Ricky's house tonight?

PARENT: No, you have to be up early for soccer practice tomorrow.

CHILD: *(Whining)* Oh, come on. I promise we'll go to bed early.

PARENT: That's one.

CHILD: But that's not fair. I never get to spend the night just because of stupid soccer.

PARENT: That's two.

CHILD: You never let me do anything! This place is like a prison. *(Kicks couch.)*

PARENT: That's three—take five.

In addition to allowing you to intervene quickly, this approach gives the child a chance (actually, two chances) to control his own behavior. And if you adhere to Dr. Phelan's no-talking rule, you can avoid what he calls "the reasoning trap."

■ **Don't yell and scream.** Ranting and raving won't get your point across more effectively. In fact, research comparing the effects of two kinds of negative consequences on the behavior of ADHD children show that exactly the opposite is true: a so-called "prudent" approach (calm, concrete, and consistent) was more effective than an approach the investigators termed "imprudent" (ignoring misbehavior too long, then responding inconsistently and in a loud, emotionally upset fashion). With the "imprudent" approach, the children's behavior deteriorated so dramatically that although this phase of the research was very brief, ethical concerns prevented the investigators from extending it!

Point Programs and Token Economies

Many professionals who use behavioral strategies with ADHD children suggest the use of point programs and "token economy" systems in which the child earns points, chips, or tokens of some kind to "purchase" privileges and access to things he enjoys. A particular advantage of point programs is that consequences, in the form of giving or taking away points, can be delivered on the spot regardless of where or when the behavior occurs. An additional advantage is that since a point cost can be negotiated for virtually any kind of reinforcer, the list of potential reinforcers is enormous. This also means that reinforcers can be varied with ease, an important point in working with ADHD children, who tend to tire of things and become bored more quickly than other children.

Point programs, however, are not for everyone because they require a considerable amount of organization and follow-through on the part of parents—requirements a parent who is struggling with his or her own ADHD might find impossible to meet. Remember that token economies were originally developed to help patients in psychiatric hospitals. In those settings, behavior can be monitored closely and access to privileges strictly controlled. In the home setting, it's much more difficult to restrict a child's access to snacks, TV, and the like, particularly in single-parent families and families in which both parents work outside the home.

For these reasons, think twice before you set up a complicated point program as a means of managing day-to-day behavior. Instead, think about reserving point programs for specific problem behavior that needs special attention.

Jeremy desperately wanted a very expensive skateboard. His parents, equally desperate to see him succeed in school, negotiated a point program based on completing homework assignments. Jeremy could earn two points daily by bringing home a sheet initialed by his teacher indicating homework was completed and turned in. If he earned all possible points during a school week, he could "rent" the skateboard for the following week. Otherwise, the skateboard would be locked in the closet for a week.

The program worked to everyone's satisfaction. During the entire school year, Jeremy only failed twice to earn the use of his beloved skateboard. His parents were pleased with his grades and Jeremy himself seemed proud of his good report cards.

In school, of course, the situation is quite different from that in the average home. Point programs and token economies are particularly suited to the school setting because:

- Daily routines and schedules are clear and generally unchanging;
- The child is under close adult supervision during most of the day;
- Access to reinforcers such as free time can be strictly controlled.

In fact, token economies and point programs are now widely used in special classrooms and special schools across the country. By completing their work, following classroom rules, and interacting appropriately with peers and teachers, children in these classrooms can earn access to a variety of privileges, such as using the computer or working with special art material.

The Bottom Line

A great deal of research has shown that behavioral methods can be useful with a broad array of behavior at home and in school—everything from helping a child increase time on task to reducing sibling squabbles. However, as we might suspect, behavioral methods are usually not as successful with problems that stem from the ADHD child's impulsivity—problems such as darting out into traffic or impulsively hitting an annoying peer.

Nor is behavior therapy a panacea. Like stimulant medication, behavior therapy techniques don't "cure" ADHD: they are a means of managing some of the problems associated with ADHD and, like stimulant medication, the effects do not last if the treatment is stopped.

In short, this is not a one-shot strategy. It requires time, organizational skills, and ongoing commitment. If you're going to embark on a behavior management program with your ADHD child, be prepared to put forth the necessary effort and do it right. An excellent guide to help you in such an endeavor is Dr. Russell Barkley's book *Taking Charge of ADHD.**

Postscript: Controversial Treatments for ADHD

What Are Controversial Treatments?

So-called "controversial treatments" are those that have been touted as helpful in treating ADHD but have not met rigorous scientific tests to determine their effectiveness. Some controversial treatments amount to little more than outright fraud; others seem to be the product of wishful thinking on the part of well-intentioned individuals who sincerely want to help ADHD children. Some, such as the concept of "remote depossession" (a therapist drives demons out of a patient who is not even present) are pretty far out there, while others, such as EEG biofeedback, seem to be reasonable in terms of theoretical underpinnings but have yet to show real clinical effectiveness.

A separate chapter could easily be devoted to this topic—indeed, Sam Goldstein and I became so engrossed in researching the subject that we wrote an entire book on it.† We reviewed an exhaustive array of controversial treatments, including:

- Controlled diets (sugar free, additive free, and nonallergenic)
- Megavitamin and mineral supplements
- Anti-motion-sickness pills, antifungal medications, amino acids, and essential fatty acids
- EEG biofeedback, cognitive therapy, sensory integrative therapy, and optometric vision training
- Chiropractic approach, Irlen lenses, osteopathic treatment.

We concluded that not a single one of these treatment approaches met scientifically acceptable standards to be considered effective in treating

---

* New York: Guilford Press, 1995.

† *Attention Deficit Disorder and Learning Disabilities: Realities, Myths and Controversial Treatments.*

ADHD or learning disabilities. And, to the present, no new evidence has appeared that would cause us to rethink our position concerning any of these approaches, nor is there supporting data for some of the treatments that have cropped up more recently. These include the herbal remedy Pycnogenol (a grape seed extract), the concoction known as "God's Recipe" (a combination that includes minerals, a grape seed extract in combination with other herbs, and multienzyme capsules), and the organic sulfur known as "MSM" (methylsulfonylmethane).

Parents as Consumers

Because I've spent so many hours poring over literature on controversial treatments, the subject is a bit old hat for me and I'm always a little surprised when a patient or conference participant asks my opinion about one of these approaches. I have to remind myself that proponents of these approaches are still putting out books and papers and giving talks to audiences that include parents of ADHD children—parents who are desperately seeking help for their child's difficulties and who are, therefore, vulnerable.

As the parent of an ADHD child, you, too, are vulnerable: wouldn't it be fantastic if there were a simple, natural substance or a training program that would make troublesome ADHD symptoms disappear? But vulnerable doesn't have to mean gullible. You owe it to yourself and to your child to be a wise consumer. Even treatments that don't have the potential for outright harm can be expensive, time-consuming, and ultimately demoralizing. Before you embark on a treatment approach that is out of what is generally considered to be the mainstream, consult with a mental health professional who is knowledgeable about ADHD.

CHAPTER 7

TREATING ASSOCIATED PROBLEMS

Overview: Then and Now

Then: A decade ago, ADHD youngsters were known to have sleep problems and problems with bowel and bladder control. It was known, too, that many ADHD children had other problems, such as impulsive lying and stealing and significant difficulty getting along with other children. Treatment programs for some of these problems were already established; others were still in their infancy.

Now: The most promising advances appear to be in monitoring and addressing the effects of sleep disturbance, an area to which many scientists have begun to devote attention, and in the area of social skills training and treatment.

Effective treatments for bowel and bladder problems are now widely known to pediatricians, who can step in quickly to treat them. Treatment approaches for lying and stealing have not changed: what has changed is our awareness that these problems need to be treated quickly, since they often signal a developing conduct disorder.

Sleep Problems

As many a weary parent can attest, sleep problems are common in young-sters with ADHD. Bedtime battles, in fact, rival homework wars as the number one source of friction in many families with an ADHD child, since these youngsters often resist bedtime with the ferocity of a cat resisting a bath.

> "Mornings are crazy at our house, but bedtimes are even worse. By eight o'clock, I've had it. All I want to do is flop on the couch for a few minutes and just stare into space. The *last* thing I want to do is chase Jason around the house, yelling at him to get in bed and stay in bed. But that's what it takes, almost every single night."

Sleep problems may be present from the earliest days of the child's life, and getting the infant to sleep can be just the first of many struggles to come. Some parents describe desperate measures, such as driving the child around the neighborhood during the wee hours to lull him to sleep. Others have almost literally stumbled, bleary-eyed, across unusual but effective methods of soothing squalling children into slumber: one mother, for example, found that her child would fall asleep in a matter of minutes if placed in an infant-carrier atop a running clothes dryer. (While this is not an energy-saving tactic in terms of the environment, it is certainly efficient in terms of conserving parental sanity.)

Like ADHD itself, sleep problems may not be outgrown with age. For many ADHD children, difficulty falling asleep remains a problem through childhood and adolescence. Ironically, the stimulant medication that helps so many ADHD youngsters function successfully during the day can result in insomnia in children who were otherwise good sleepers, and a worsening of insomnia already present in others.

Many ADHD children also awaken during the night and have diffi-culty returning to sleep. Some are frequent visitors to the parental bed and, when denied access, may actually "camp out" on the floor or out-side the bedroom door. Pronounced aversion to sleeping alone is *not* typical of ADHD youngsters: instead, it may signal a mood disorder or an anxiety disorder, since interrupted sleep is common in both conditions.

Even ADHD children who do not actively resist bedtime or wander the house at night can suffer from sleep deprivation, unbeknownst to their parents. Although restless sleep has long been considered characteristic of ADHD children, it is only recently that we have learned that thrashing and jerking about during sleep can interfere with sleep so much that sleep deprivation results.[141]

Sleep apnea, a condition in which the upper airway is blocked during sleep, might play a role in attentional and behavioral problems.[142] A common cause of sleep apnea in children is enlarged tonsils or adenoids which prevent the child from breathing freely during sleep. As the child struggles to breathe, he may snore loudly and thrash about, so sleep quality is poor and the child is, in effect, sleep deprived. Because ADHD children often have problems with respiratory infections, they may be at particular risk for sleep apnea.

Since ADHD often coexists with conduct disorder, it is not surprising to find that conduct-disordered youngsters have sleep-related complaints similar to those of ADHD youngsters. Sleep disturbances are also particularly common among individuals with Tourette's syndrome: unlike youngsters with ADHD, however, patients with Tourette's often have night terrors and sleepwalking, problems that are not seen with particular frequency among ADHD individuals.[143]

Some researchers believe that the sleep problems of ADHD youngsters can exacerbate symptoms of ADHD. In individuals of any age, loss of sleep results in irritability and poor frustration tolerance, difficulty concentrating, mood swings, and forgetfulness. (Think about it: how do *you* feel after a night with little sleep?) There are actually cases on record in which people with severe sleep disorders were incorrectly diagnosed as suffering from psychiatric disorders, so serious were the behavioral and emotional consequences of sleep deprivation.

Treating the Problem

If you suspect that a sleep disorder complicates your child's already-difficult behavior, what should you do? Begin by ruling out a medical cause for the problem, since serous otitis media, gastroesophageal reflux, and allergies to cow's milk can cause significant sleep problems in infants and toddlers.

If no medical cause is found, establish an age-appropriate sleep schedule and stick to that schedule, no matter how much your child protests. Don't deviate from the schedule, even on weekends, until you are sure that the problem has been identified and resolved, and don't give your child any food or beverage containing caffeine (such as caffeinated soda or chocolate). These measures are difficult to enforce, but in some cases they will produce good improvement in sleep quality, with corresponding improvement in daytime behavior.

If this doesn't solve the problem, the next step is to observe your child and record your observations in a sleep log over a period of a month or so. If your child has difficulty falling asleep, quietly check on him at fifteen-minute intervals to determine how long it takes him to fall asleep. If you believe that snoring or restless sleep is the problem, plan to spend a few nights observing your child for a few minutes out of every hour for as long as you can remain awake.

Then make an appointment with the medical or mental health professional who is most familiar with your child to review your observations, discuss the problem, and decide on a plan of action. The professional might recommend a consultation with a neurologist who specializes in diagnosing and treating sleep problems if he thinks there is a need for further evaluation. Alternatively, the professional might suggest a specific intervention, such as medication.

Medication. Various medications are helpful in treating sleep problems associated with ADHD. These medications do *not* include sleeping pills or tranquilizers, medications that seldom have a place in the treatment of childhood sleep disturbances. Instead, the physician might recommend a trial of clonidine, which has been shown to be helpful in treating sleep disturbances in youngsters with ADHD and youngsters with Tourette's syndrome (see Chapter 5). For children with coexisting mood or anxiety disorders, a tricyclic antidepressant such as imipramine may be prescribed at bedtime to help with both mood/anxiety and sleep. Trazadone, a sedating antidepressant often used to treat depression-related sleep problems in adults, has also been used for this purpose in children, although its use in children has not been well studied.

Melatonin, a hormone manufactured by the pineal gland, plays an important role in regulating the sleep-wake cycle, and some studies have shown that it helps insomnia in adults.[144] Reports that it is helpful with insomnia in children have also appeared[145] but there are no controlled studies. Since melatonin is available in health food stores as a dietary supplement, some people consider it "natural" and therefore safe. But, in fact, the melatonin found in health food stores is chemically synthesized and may contain a variety of impurities and herbal preparations. Therefore, *it would be wise to await the results of further research before using melatonin.*

Alternative Treatments. Behavioral methods such as progressive relaxation and cognitive therapy may be of mild benefit to some youngsters with insomnia and with fears that interfere with sleep. If these approaches are used, it's important that they be combined with other sleep-hygiene measures such as a strictly enforced sleep schedule and removal of caffeine from the diet.

In our clinic, we have used a technique known as "dawn-dusk simulation" to help ADHD youngsters who suffer from insomnia. This approach uses a rheostat attached to an ordinary bedside lamp. The device,★ when set for the desired bedtime, gradually dims the light from full brightness to full dark over the course of forty-five minutes, thereby mimicking natural dusk. In the morning, the reverse occurs: the light gradually brightens, mimicking natural dawn. Clinical reports indicate that this approach, which seems to "reset" the sleep cycle, can be helpful with people who have difficulty falling asleep and waking up in the morning.

Wetting and Soiling

As if their other problems were not enough to shatter the self-esteem of ADHD youngsters, many have problems with bowel and bladder control long beyond the age at which other children have gained control of these bodily functions. Why this is the case is unknown at present: perhaps

---

★ The device, known as SunUp, is available from the SunBox Company, 19217 Orbit Drive, Gaithersburg, MD 20879–4149 (1-800-548-3968).

bladder problems reflect a general neurological "immaturity," as some have speculated. Bowel problems may be more common in picky eaters whose diets lack sufficient fiber to keep the bowel functioning properly. Regardless of the cause, however, we need to take steps to help these children gain control of bowel and bladder functions.

Wetting (Enuresis)

Bed-wetting, sometimes lasting into the teen years, is particularly common in ADHD children.[146] Daytime wetting is less common, especially in older children, and may signal organic complications.[147] Enuretic children have to urinate more frequently than children without such problems, and they are less sensitive to signals from their bladder indicating a need to urinate.

Only in about ten percent of enuretic children is there a medical reason for the problem and, when there is, other symptoms usually appear, such as dribbling or painful urination. Nevertheless, any child who wets should have a physical examination and a urinalysis because enuretic children, especially girls, are prone to urinary tract infections.[148] These must be treated, although the wetting may still have to be treated when the infection has been eliminated.

Daytime Wetting. Some ADHD children wet because they are reluctant to interrupt their play for something as mundane as going to the bathroom. With these children, pair a reward program with positive practice: if the child is dry through the day, he earns a small reward in the evening. If he has an accident, however, he must "practice" appropriate toilet behavior as soon afterward as possible. For example, if the accident occurred while he was playing in the yard, he should walk quickly from the yard to the bathroom and go through the motions of urinating, then return to the yard and start over. Ten repetitions of this procedure should follow every accident.

If this method is not helpful, or if your child has accidents at times other than when he is "too busy" to go to the bathroom, he might have poor sphincter control and/or a bladder that contracts very strongly when only small amounts of urine are present. The following program can be helpful with both problems:

■ For three days, record the time of day and the amount each time the child urinates. (Have the child urinate into a clear plastic measuring cup marked in units of $1/2$ ounce—and be prepared for lots of giggles with this one!) Record the greatest amount of urine and use that as the goal to be beaten on the fourth day.

■ On the fourth day, tell the child that each time he feels the urge to urinate, he should hold off as long as he can. This will train his bladder to hold more so the amount will be greater when he finally urinates. If he beats his previous record when he urinates, he will earn stickers, stars, or points toward a treat.

■ Each time the child urinates, he should practice starting and stopping the stream of urine to strengthen sphincter muscles controlling urination. (Again, be prepared for giggles.)

■ Encourage your child to drink more (noncaffeinated) fluids during the day so that he has more opportunities to practice the steps above. Explain that this will help his bladder get bigger and stronger.

Continue the program until daytime wetting is no longer a problem. This usually happens by the time the child is consistently able to hold about ten to fourteen ounces per voiding.

Bed-wetting. Although bed-wetting is a fairly common problem among children, for the ADHD child who is in constant conflict with his environment and whose self-esteem is already at rock bottom, bed-wetting is just one more failure in a long series of failures.

Aaron wanted to die when his sister told her friends that he wet the bed. It was hard enough to pretend that he didn't care about failing so many tests in school or that Mrs. August always yelled at him for daydreaming in class. It was especially hard to act as if he didn't care when he was the last one chosen to play kickball at recess and to ignore snickers and taunts when he tripped or missed the ball.

But this—oh, man, this was too much! He knew the other fifth-graders would be merciless when the word got around. Brian Gavin would get all the others to gang up—Aaron shuddered when he imagined it. "Maybe," he thought, "if I pray real hard, I won't be wet when I wake up tomorrow." But he knew it wouldn't work. Nothing else had worked. Even his parents had finally given up and just tried to act like it didn't matter. It did, though: he could tell by the look on his mother's face each time she changed his wet sheets.

Before you begin a program to help with bed-wetting, assure your child that wetting doesn't mean that he is bad or lazy. Tell him, too, that he isn't alone: in a class of thirty first- or second-graders, three or four still bed-wet and, in the average fourth- or fifth-grade classroom, two children still have the problem.

The most successful method for treating bed-wetting is the urine alarm.* Based on teaching the child to recognize and respond to bladder signals, the urine alarm consists of a moisture-sensitive pad on which the child sleeps. When the pad is moistened with urine, it triggers an alarm that awakens the child, who then goes (or is taken) to the bathroom. Eventually, the child responds to the cues of a full bladder without the assistance of the alarm.

With the urine alarm, eighty to ninety percent of children achieve dryness after five to twelve weeks of treatment. Relapses do occur, but usually respond quickly when the alarm is reintroduced. "Overlearning" seems to enhance results and prevent relapses, so the more opportunities the child has to practice, the better. Opportunities to practice can be increased by increasing the child's fluid intake in the early evening. A reward program will also help by keeping motivation high.

Behavioral programs like the urine alarm are the treatment of choice in managing bed-wetting. If behavioral programs fail, however, or if there is a need to institute emergency measures so that a child can attend camp or go on an extended family trip, medication can be useful. The antidepressant medication imipramine (Tofranil) is often prescribed in relatively low doses (usually 10 to 75 milligrams) although some children need higher doses.[149] In most cases, there is an immediate reduction in the frequency of wetting, although only about one-third achieve total dryness. Some children who have an immediate positive response develop tolerance to the medication after two to six weeks, and frequency of wetting again increases.

Administered as a nasal spray, desmopressin (DDAVP) has recently become the medication of choice among some physicians. Used for many

---

* The urine alarm is available from stores like Montgomery Ward and Sears, Roebuck.

years to treat children with diabetes insipidus, it is considered safe and it appears to be at least as effective as imipramine.[150]

Medication is *not* a cure for bed-wetting: when medication is stopped, bed-wetting occurs again almost immediately. As noted, however, medication can be useful on an occasional basis for events like sleepovers and camp or as a last resort for the child who has not been helped by other methods.

Soiling (Encopresis)

As the nurse ushered them into Dr. Benson's office, Mrs. French had to practically drag nine-year-old Timothy. "Tim, you don't look happy to be here today," Dr. Benson remarked. Tim looked at the doctor and shook his head. "Tell the doctor why you're here," his mother instructed. Tim hung his head and remained silent. "Tell her," his mother repeated. "You know why you're here." Tim only shook his head. Mrs. French made it clear to her son that he had stretched her patience to the limit. Through clenched teeth she insisted, "You *do* know why you're here. Now tell the doctor what you do." Tim kept his head down so they couldn't see the glisten of tears. In a small voice he admitted, "I poop in my pants."

Soiling, which is more common in boys than in girls, usually occurs in the late afternoon or evening and stress seems to increase the likelihood of occurrence. Some children pass large stools in their pants or in other inappropriate places, while others pass only small amounts which appear as stains or smears in their underwear. Because soiling may wax and wane, parents conclude that it is deliberate: "He's controlled it before, so he ought to be able to do it all the time," they assume.

As toddlers, many children who soil are reluctant to use the toilet for bowel movements and may cry, cling, or throw tantrums if efforts are made to force them. Since the history of these children usually reveals at least one episode of constipation resulting in a painful bowel movement, it is likely that they have learned to fear the toilet, with the result that they struggle to withhold stool to avoid anticipated pain.

Unfortunately, withholding results in a distended bowel, impacted feces, and relaxed anal sphincter muscles. In severe cases, a leakage of watery stool around the impaction can mimic diarrhea. When the bowel is distended for long periods of time, the child is no longer sensitive to signals from the colon and rectum indicating the need to have a bowel movement. This is why children who soil often insist "I didn't know I needed to go," which seems incomprehensible to parents.

Soiling is actually quite easy to treat, as most pediatricians now know. In several studies, success rates in the neighborhood of eighty to one hundred percent are reported, a figure consistent with my own findings. In my practice, I've had excellent results with a program that consists of a bowel cleanout, education, explanation, and retraining.

Step One: Explanation and Education. The child who soils needs to know that his problem is due to a physical condition. To explain the physical problem, draw a circle within a larger circle. The outer circle represents muscles that move waste material through the inner part of the tube. Waste sometimes accumulates in the inner tube if the child is too busy to go to the bathroom or if his diet doesn't contain the right things to keep waste moving along the tube. When unmoved waste accumulates, it blocks the tube and causes it to bulge. This makes the muscles of the intestinal wall thin and weak, so they can't make the waste move along the tube.

Tell your child that you are going to help him build up the muscles in his intestinal walls and that he can learn to control his bowel movements as these muscles get stronger. Explain that the first step is to get rid of the bulge that is currently blocking his intestines so that he can get off to a good start on his "muscle-training program."

Step Two: Bowel Cleanout. Get a medical evaluation to rule out the possibility of an organic cause before beginning a bowel cleanout regimen of enemas, laxatives, and suppositories. It usually takes about two to three weeks of such a regimen to be certain that no waste is retained. Your pediatrician can guide you in this process.

Step Three: Retraining. A retraining program involves the following:

- Set a time for toileting each day (preferably twenty to thirty minutes after a meal). Set daily consequences for performance and nonperformance. Elaborate rewards are not necessary: the child can simply earn television time or computer time. If you use money as a reward, you should also impose a fine for failure, since ADHD youngsters can often be motivated by "double-or-nothing" challenges.

- Verify reports of success. The mere sound of a toilet flushing is not sufficient: you need visual proof.
- If your child does not have a bowel movement for two consecutive days, use a suppository so that the impaction process doesn't begin again.
- Give your child a high-fiber diet, including bran cereals, bran muffins, whole-grain breads, salads, and raw vegetables.

This program usually produces excellent results within the first week or so. If relapses occur, they can usually be treated with careful surveillance of diet and regular toilet habits.

Note, however, that young children who are reluctant to use the toilet must be helped to overcome their fear before a retraining program can be started. For children who are very fearful and become greatly upset at the prospect of using the toilet, seek professional assistance to help the child overcome his fear.

Lying and Stealing

Lying

"I'm at the end of my rope with that kid. He knows I can't stand a liar. After all the times I've punished him for lying, you'd think he would finally learn. But, no! Even when you've got the proof right there in front of him, he'll still lie until he's blue in the face. I just don't understand why he does it, when he knows how crazy it makes me."

Like the rest of us, children lie because they fear disapproval or punishment for misdeeds. And, like us, they may also lie to avoid unpleasant tasks or chores.

Lying to Avoid Punishment. Lying to avoid punishment is particularly likely if a child is often subjected to expectations he cannot meet—a situation in which the ADHD child frequently finds himself. The likelihood of self-protective lying is even greater if the child expects to receive harsh punishment for his misdeeds and transgressions.

To emphasize the value of truthfulness, some parents tell their children that if they lie about a misdeed they will be punished twice, once for the misdeed and once for lying about it. On the face of it, this approach makes sense, but there are problems with it. Suppose your child confesses his misdeed: if you punish him, you are in the awkward position of punishing your child for telling the truth. On the other hand, if you do not impose a punishment, you are in effect telling the child, "It's okay to break the rules as long as you tell the truth about it."

This tactic also tempts a child to play double-or-nothing. "If I admit it, I'll be punished for sure," your child may reason. "If I lie, I might be punished twice as hard, but I *might* get away with the lie and avoid any punishment altogether." For ADHD children, especially, this gamble is often irresistible since many are impulsive risk-takers who seldom think about consequences before they act. This is particularly likely to be the case if there is any uncertainty about the consequences ("Maybe they won't find out").

Parents sometimes unintentionally tempt a child to lie by the way in which they confront him. To a child, the question "Did you break the lamp?" may sound like a genuine request for information, implying that you really have no idea who broke the lamp. In such a situation, the temptation to lie is almost too much for any child to resist.

As noted above, we are *all* tempted to lie when asked to incriminate ourselves. Why, then, should we insist that a child testify against himself by demanding a confession from him? A more sensible approach would be to gather all the facts from other sources and make a decision based on this evidence.

But what if it is not clear whether your child is guilty? All parents sometimes find themselves in the role of Grand Inquisitor when they suspect that a child has broken a rule but are reluctant to punish him unfairly. Remember, decisions in this imperfect world can't always be based on absolute certainty. Lacking evidence, it is probably better to avoid the issue and forgo discipline. However, if the evidence clearly points to your child as the culprit, impose a penalty. While your child may occasionally be punished unfairly, you can be sure that these occasions will be more than offset by the number of times he manages to avoid detection and gets off with no penalty for misdeeds he does commit. (Remember your own childhood and how the tally came out?)

If your child attempts to cover up a misdeed by lying, don't get drawn into a game of "courtroom" ("You know you did it." "No, honest, I didn't do it"). Instead, impose a penalty for lying (work penalties are well suited to this purpose) and bring the discussion to an abrupt close. Later, when neither of you is upset, you and your child should discuss the importance of honesty among family members.

Lying to Avoid Unpleasant Tasks. Hyperactive children often lie to avoid unpleasant tasks and chores:

- "I took a shower (. . . I just didn't use any soap or water)",
- "I did put gas in the car (. . . last month)";
- "Yes, I walked the dog (. . . yesterday)";
- "I don't have any homework tonight (. . . it's not due until tomorrow)."

Lies like these are crazy-making to parents because they seem so senseless. "Why does he do it?" they ask. "He knows he can't get away with it. He knows he's going to be caught." And, indeed, he will be caught—just as soon as the dog soils the rug an hour later or the teacher calls for his homework at nine A.M. the next day.

Even though unpleasant consequences are certain to follow, they may not seem real to an ADHD child since they are not immediate. To the child who lies to avoid doing his homework, for example, tomorrow is a long way away and—who knows—maybe the teacher will get sick or forget to ask for the homework or maybe the school will blow up or the world will end before tomorrow morning.

Parents are also bewildered by the lengths to which some ADHD children will go to avoid boring tasks. The child who carefully wets his toothbrush and leaves the toothpaste tube sitting on the sink but doesn't actually brush his teeth is a good example. My own favorite example is the youngster (my sister, in fact) who was told to vacuum the living room carpet while her parents went out for a few hours. Rather than fetch the vacuum from the hall closet, she worked her way across every inch of the large room, brushing up the nap of the carpet with her foot to give it a freshly vacuumed appearance. This method took at least ten times longer than it would have taken to simply vacuum the rug in conventional fashion. "But," as she later explained, "vacuuming is so *boring*."

How can you cope with a child who lies to avoid tasks and chores? Forewarned is forearmed: it's safer to *assume* that the ADHD child will try to dodge dull tasks. This means that close supervision rather than an honor system should be the rule, at least in situations which parents know are particularly difficult. In other words:

DON'T ASK: "Did you clean your room?"
INSTEAD: Set a regular time for daily room inspection. Post a list in the child's room of tasks to be accomplished by inspection time (e.g., bed made, clothes hanging on hooks or hangers in closet, etc.).

DON'T ASK: "Did you practice the piano today?"
INSTEAD: Have the child practice while you are at home, even if you are in another room. If you can't be there, have the child make a tape recording of daily practice sessions. Then listen to the tape while you're in the car or working out on the treadmill.

DON'T ASK: "Do you have homework tonight?"
INSTEAD: Have the child's teacher initial the child's assignment book daily (see Chapter 8). This way, you can be certain about what homework was assigned.

Stealing

Most young children experiment with stealing. Fortunately, most respond to the time-honored practice of being marched back to the scene of the crime, under parental escort, to return the stolen goods and apologize to the victim. By the age of six or so, most children have learned to curb their impulses and refrain from stealing.

Certainly, not all ADHD children steal. Many—probably the majority—respect the property rights of others. As a group, however, ADHD children are more vulnerable to temptation than other children, for several reasons:

- **Poor impulse control.** Some impulsive ADHD youngsters cannot resist the temptation to help themselves to other people's property. (Note: stimulant medication is often useful in helping children who steal on impulse but is probably of little value for children who methodically work out plans in advance of stealing.)

- **Uncertain consequences.** If there are no witnesses on the scene, the potential consequences of stealing may seem remote or nonexistent: "How can I get caught if no one sees me?"

- **Low self-esteem and poor social skills.** Children sometimes steal to compensate for a lack of positive things in their lives, such as affection, friendship, and respect for their abilities. Some give away the stolen goods in an attempt to impress peers and buy friendship.

Treating the Problem. Parents are right to be worried about a child who habitually steals. At best, the child will earn a reputation as a thief; at worst, he will end up in juvenile court. If your child habitually steals, take action now.

- **Don't minimize the problem.** It may be so hard for you to acknowledge that your child steals that you use euphemisms such as "take" and "borrow" when talking about his stealing. Remember though, whether it is a quarter from your purse or a sweater from a department store, stealing is stealing.

- **Discuss the problem calmly.** Don't yell, threaten, or give a sermon. Tell your child why you're so concerned—that other people won't trust him; that he'll lose friends; and that he'll pay a high price in many other ways for stealing. Point out, too, how bad people feel when they lose something of value to them.

- **Establish clear rules and penalties.** Don't allow the child to bring home "gifts" and things he has "found." Consider all such items stolen, confiscate them, and impose a penalty.

- **Provide supervision.** Many young thieves are "wanderers" who have much unsupervised time. Children who habitually steal need close supervision, including room checks and even pocket searches, until you are sure the problem has been corrected. This approach may be distasteful to you, but support and prevention are much better than punishment after the fact.

"Nobody Likes Me!"

In her own words, Nancy was a "social outcast." In preschool, she was quiet and standoffish and usually played alone instead of joining the other children in games and fantasy play. In elementary school, her disheveled appearance, messy desk, and learning problems made her a target for nicknames like "Nancy the Nerd." She was teased, too, about the "babyish" toys she brought to school and about her lack of skills in sports and playground games.

The children in Nancy's neighborhood seldom included her in their activities and she spent much of her time in front of the television. When the girl next door invited Nancy to her birthday party, she made it clear that the invitation was issued only because her parents insisted. Nancy had a miserable time at the party and returned home in tears.

Not all ADHD children have problems like Nancy's. The ADHD child with a sunny disposition, for example, may have no trouble finding friends, even if he is loud and boisterous. Or, if an ADHD child is respected for his athletic skills, his peers may accept his bossiness as "leadership." Occasionally, fate intervenes and the ADHD child gets lucky, but often the opposite is true.

No one in the neighborhood could keep up with Jeffrey—no one, that is, until Edward moved in down the street. Like Jeffrey, Edward had boundless energy. After racing their bikes through the neighborhood all morning and swimming all afternoon (if they weren't thrown out of the pool), both were ready for a wild game of badminton after supper. In addition to endless energy, both boys had hot tempers, so loud arguments often punctuated their play, but the squabbles blew over as quickly as they had begun. Most often, they were a team, united in plotting diabolical new ways to torment Jeffrey's older brother or Edward's older sister.

Unlike Jeffrey, many ADHD children do not have the good fortune of finding a boon companion, and the same qualities that bring them into

conflict with adults cause them to have problems in their relationships
with other children. Some seem completely unaware of the subtle cues
and signals that regulate social exchanges. In a conversation between two
people, for example, words carry only about a third of the total "message." The rest is conveyed through nonverbal signals like eye contact,
facial expression, and gesture. A person who fails to detect these crucial
signals is likely to be thought eccentric, self-centered, and boorish. Failing to detect that others are bored or annoyed, he may talk too much,
carry a joke too far, or insist on continuing an activity long after others in
the group have tired of it.

There are other reasons, too, for the social problems of ADHD children. Some, like the little girl described above, are awkward, spacey, and
socially "out of it." Others, particularly those with coexisting anxiety
disorders, are almost pathologically shy and withdrawn and tend to avoid
any interaction with peers. If a child is also clumsy on the athletic field
and struggles with learning disabilities in the classroom, he has few if any
opportunities to achieve acceptance and approval from peers, so the child
is simply neglected and ignored. Although some of these children may
become recluses as adults, most find or make a social niche for themselves
as they grow older.

On the other hand, the social problems of impulsive, aggressive
ADHD children often worsen over time, sometimes to such a point that
the child is actively victimized and assaulted by other children. The problems of these children frequently begin in the early preschool years and
stem not so much from their hyperactivity as from their impulsive and
aggressive behavior such as shoving, grabbing or throwing objects, insulting or threatening others, and intentionally interfering with the activities
of others (e.g., knocking over a block tower constructed by others). Research[151,152] has shown that other children may not retaliate at first but,
over time, they not only react with counteraggression—they begin to
engage in unprovoked taunting, teasing, and attacks on the ADHD child.
The child retaliates in turn and the cycle escalates.

Unfortunately, once this cycle is set in motion, it tends to perpetuate
itself. Peers, having learned to expect the worst from the child, view all
his behavior with a jaundiced eye. Thus, they tend to disregard any
instances of positive, prosocial behavior but react with hostility to
even minor offenses they would overlook in another, more popular

child. They continue to treat him poorly and, when he retaliates, his behavior only further serves to confirm their view of him as a "bad egg."

Once a child's negative reputation is established within a group, simply changing the child's behavior through such means as medication and social skills training may not be enough to change his reputation. It may also be necessary to modify the way his peers see him. How can this be done?

Treating the Problem

If your ADHD child has a hard time making friends, you've shared the pain of his social isolation. You've probably experienced a host of other emotions too: impatience with the child for being so inept socially; helpless rage at peers who taunt and tease; and a nagging worry that he will never find friends or fit in. No doubt you've tried to help: how often have you counseled, "Just ignore them when they tease you"? How many times have you advised, "Don't be so bossy. The other kids don't like it"?

It's a safe bet that your efforts have met with little success. What else can you do? Might social skills training help? Maybe—maybe not. Many of these programs focus on teaching prosocial behavior, such as how to greet another child, pay a compliment, and ask another child to play. But such skills will be of little use to the ADHD child who is too timid and anxious to actually use them or to a rejected child whose attempts will probably be rebuffed by peers. (This explains why many social skills programs for ADHD children have met with only limited success.)

Instead of a one-size-fits-all approach to treating the social problems of ADHD children, we need programs that are very carefully tailored to meet the needs of the individual child. Obviously, we can't design a program to meet the needs of a particular child unless we know exactly what his needs are—in this situation, as in the case of ADHD itself, we again see that it is crucial to do a careful evaluation before leaping headlong into treatment.

Helping the Shy or Awkward ADHD Child. Shy children often hang back from socializing with peers because they fear that others will ridicule them if they make a mistake. In some cases, professional intervention may be necessary to help the child deal with paralyzing anxiety.

In other cases, however, a child's social life can be helped by improving his play skills. If, for example, your child doesn't know the rules of the games his peers like to play, teach him or find someone who can. If he lacks the necessary skills—if he is poorly coordinated and can't throw or catch a ball, jump rope, or ride a bike, practice with him. If you lack the skill or the patience, look into programs that teach the fundamentals of running, throwing, catching, dribbling, and passing in a noncompetitive setting. If no such programs are available in your area, consider hiring a "personal trainer" to help your child learn these skills.

Look for other activities, too, that will give your child a feeling of mastery and accomplishment and that will bring him into contact with other people. Lessons of almost any kind are great for this purpose, and the list is as long as your imagination: painting, dancing, tennis, karate, golf, guitar, fencing, skating, acting, horseback riding, and so on. Church youth groups and scouting can also be helpful, especially if you become a den parent, a scoutmaster, or a youth group leader.

Helping the Aggressive/Rejected ADHD Child. Programs for these children must be multifaceted because there are many problems to address. The impulsive behavior that is so aggravating to peers is usually not amenable to treatment through behavioral methods. Instead, it is more efficiently addressed through medication.

What you can do:

▪ **Teach and encourage prosocial behavior.** Just treating antisocial behavior is not enough if the rejected child is also weak in the area of prosocial skills. Social skills training programs can be helpful in filling this void—if, indeed, the child really lacks the know-how—something that should be determined before trying to teach skills the child might already possess but just doesn't use.

Even when a child knows the "right" thing to do or say in a situation, however, there's no guarantee that he will actually do it or say it. Sometimes, anxiety interferes and the child lapses into silly, offputting behavior. I've seen this in my office countless times: a child who is a poised, charming companion when alone with me suddenly acts goofy and annoying when his parents join us—not because his parents are a bad influence, but because the pressure of interacting with several adults causes him to lose his composure. I've found that it's helpful to label this behavior (I call it "the goofer"), identify it when it occurs, and then help the child deal with the anxiety that provokes it.

■ **Help the child interpret the behavior of others.** It's likely that rejected ADHD children will also need help in learning how to interpret the behavior of others, since many aggressive children misinterpret the intentions of others as hostile when no hostility is really intended. Again, social skills programs can help, but parents can help, too, by teaching the child to distinguish between intentional versus unintentional transgressions of others. If, for example, your child is working on a complicated construction project with building toys and another child walks over and kicks the structure into ruins, you might say, "I certainly agree that it was mean of T.J. to have done that. I think you should tell him that it was mean and that it made you angry." On the other hand, if the damage was accidental—T.J. wasn't paying any attention to where he was walking— point this out: "T.J. was in a hurry and wasn't looking where he was going. I know that he should have been more careful and I know you're upset. Why don't you ask T.J. if he'll help you fix it?"

■ **Modify how others see your child.** Even after all these pieces have been put in place, however, the child must still contend with a bad reputation and how it affects the way other children see him. How can you change the way other children see your child?

By planning activities that children enjoy and inviting a classmate or a neighbor child to go along, you can pave the way for others to begin to see your child in a more positive light. Trips to the theater, amusement parks, and sports events are fun for children, as are swimming parties, sleepovers, movies, and dinner at your child's favorite fast-food restaurant. Steer away from competitive activities, since many ADHD children become overaroused and out of control when they compete. Instead, provide cooperative games* and plan cooperative activities in which the children work together toward a common goal—activities such as building models, assembling a craft project, going on a scavenger hunt, and the like. Research has shown that engaging in cooperative activities is a particularly powerful way to foster liking of participants for one another.

Before each event, discuss the plans in detail with your child to avoid

---

* Catalogue available from Family Pastimes, RR 4, Perth, Ontario, Canada, K7H 3C6.

potential pitfalls. Explain, too, how to be a good host to his guest or guests. Provide as much structure and supervision as you think your child will need, and be prepared to step in quietly and pleasantly if you're needed.

Teachers who have socially isolated hyperactive children in their classrooms can help too. In some ways, this is an easier task for a teacher than a parent because a teacher does not have to create opportunities for the child to interact with other children: in a class of thirty children, these opportunities are ready-made. Suggestions for teachers are given in Chapter 9.

CHAPTER 8

BLESS THIS HOUSE

Holding It Together on the Home Front

Overview: Then and Now

Then: A decade ago, parents of ADHD children often had nowhere to turn for help, understanding, and support. Friends, neighbors, family members—even complete strangers—felt free to offer unsolicited advice on "how to straighten that kid out." These same critics, of course, were often aghast at the idea of "drugging" a child with stimulant medication. Many parents could not even look to their spouse for comfort, and if their marriage faltered under the strain of life with an ADHD child, marriage counseling could only do so much, since the real source of stress was not addressed.

Now: Increased awareness of ADHD has resulted in increased support for parents of ADHD children. Grandparents, having read about ADHD in *Newsweek* and other popular magazines, are more enlightened, as are friends and neighbors. A nationwide network of support groups provides information, education, and mutual support to parents. With expanded knowledge of the genetics of the disorder, ADHD and related problems are now more commonly recognized and treated in parents as well as children, enabling them to function more effectively as parents and as people.

The Problems Parents Face

Life with an ADHD child is a lot like a roller-coaster ride: It's exhilarating and exciting, but it sometimes feels like your stomach drops out from under you, leaving you breathless, disoriented, and a little ill. The highs can be pretty high, it's true, but the lows can really be the proverbial pits. And unlike a roller coaster in an amusement park, you don't have any choice about going along for the ride.

Over the years, I've heard from many parents who have been passengers on the ADHD roller coaster. One of my favorite letters arrived shortly after *Your Hyperactive Child* was published ten years ago.

Dear Dr. Ingersoll:

I read your book *Your Hyperactive Child,* cover to cover in one sitting. You described my child and my family so accurately that I was sure you had hidden in a closet to watch us and collect material for your book.

Our son, Evan, is now nine years old. He takes Ritalin, which has helped a lot. We've also worked with a therapist who helped us work out a good behavior modification system, so, all in all, we're doing much better.

There were times, though, when I really thought we wouldn't make it. We've been confused by conflicting advice from professionals and we've been humiliated by Evan's wild behavior in front of family, friends, and total strangers. We've gone through guilt, wondering what we might have done wrong, and through anger, worry, and anxiety about Evan's future. Evan's problems have affected our marriage, our relationship with the neighbors—even our relationship with our dog: we finally gave our beautiful little Westie to my niece because Evan pestered her so much that if she hadn't bitten him, I would have.

Even though the worst is behind us now and Evan is doing so much better, I'll never forget what a painful, lonely struggle it has been. Even now, I sometimes wonder "Am I handling this the right way? Am I handling anything with Evan the right way? *Is* there a right way?"

As this letter so poignantly illustrates, life with an ADHD child can be hard on everyone in the family, right down to the dog! Anyone who has ever lived with an ADHD child knows that these children can be difficult, demanding, and exhausting. Their tendency to be forgetful, absent-minded, and messy causes problems in busy families in which daily schedules are planned with no time to spare. Many of these youngsters are argumentative and so skilled in the art of debating ridiculous points that a simple request to feed the dog can lead to a wrangle that only the Supreme Court could settle.

Then, too, there are the problems you face when your child's behavior brings him into conflict with people outside of the immediate family. There is shame and embarrassment when:

- He is expelled from a preschool gymnastics class because he is so rowdy and unmanageable.
- He races headlong through crowds of shoppers at the mall or throws a world-class tantrum in the grocery store.
- Other parents won't let their children play with him or invite him to birthday parties.

And there is anxiety—sometimes stark terror—if your child is a reckless daredevil who is a familiar figure in the local emergency room. There are nagging worries, too, about the future: this child can't even take out the trash without getting lost or into some kind of mischief, how will he ever manage on his own? What's going to happen to him when you're not right there, dogging his footsteps?

Finally, there is anger and resentment when, for example, you race across town for the third time in a week to retrieve his forgotten book bag before the janitor locks the school for the night. Certainly, it is frustrating to live with a child who is never where he is supposed to be or doing what he should be doing.

Sometimes, anger and resentment spill over onto others. Frustrated parents might blame an unsympathetic teacher for the child's difficulties in school. Others may complain about a coach who benches the youngster for every little infraction. Still others lash out at neighbor children for teasing the ADHD and goading him into fights. Sometimes the anger extends to other children in the family: parents may accuse them of lack of concern for their ADHD sibling, complain that they are selfish, and demand the impossible in terms of patience and understanding.

Perhaps the saddest form of misdirected anger occurs when parents, in their confusion and despair, blame each other for the child's problems. One parent (usually Dad) complains, "You're too lenient with him; you let him get away with murder." The other parent (usually Mom) counters, "You're too harsh with him. All you do is yell at him and pick on him."

Problems can be amplified if the child behaves better for one parent than for the other. In these cases, it is usually the father who elicits better behavior, because children tend to be somewhat more cooperative and less unruly with male adults. Some fathers assume that this reflects their superior parenting skills and are tactless enough to say so ("Why can't you make him behave? I never have any problems with him"). This, of course, adds insult to injury, and the battle is on!

In other ways, too, raising a child with ADHD can strain a marriage to the breaking point. When you've spent the day chasing an active child, cleaning up after him, and staving off a hundred small disasters, it's difficult to find the energy to hold your head up, let alone listen with interest and sympathy to news about your spouse's day at work. Romance, intimacy, closeness, all go by the board. And when all leisure time is spent with an ADHD child, tempers fray and arguments erupt, further eroding the marital relationship.

Other children in the family are also affected by a sibling with ADHD. Brothers and sisters resent the presence of a difficult, intrusive ADHD child who keeps the family in turmoil, spoils holidays and family outings, and demands so much attention.

> "I'd give anything if my kids could get along together. My older children say that they hate Carl, my ADHD child. I can't seem to make them understand that he has a problem and they should be more patient with him. They gripe about all the time I have to spend with him. And they're right: he takes so much of my time and energy that sometimes there just isn't much left over for them.

Finally, relationships with the extended family may suffer. Some parents of ADHD children dread large family gatherings, knowing that their child will be compared unfavorably with his cousins. Families can be split apart if relatives criticize or reject the ADHD child.

"With everything I have to deal with, it would be nice if my parents would pitch in and offer to take Eric off my hands for an afternoon. But they don't, even though they have my sister's kids over for a couple of days at a time. I guess I can understand it: they're not young anymore and Eric really is a handful. But it still hurts!"

"I know Bob's parents don't think we're doing a good job with Jessie. They don't come right out and say so, but I can tell from the way they act that they think we're pretty rotten parents. We don't visit them much anymore because I'm a nervous wreck when we do."

Coping with the Problems

Is there hope for a marriage strained by the presence of an ADHD child? What can you do to minimize sibling squabbles and outright warfare? How can you safeguard your own sanity while dealing with the needs of your ADHD child, your other children, your spouse, and all the other people who make so many demands on your time and your energy?

Let's start with how you can keep yourself sane in the midst of all the chaos around you. You are, after all, Number One, because, if you collapse, the rest of the family will be in big trouble.

Keeping Yourself Together

If you frequently find yourself on the brink of hysterics with your ADHD child, what steps should you take? If you are often furious with the child—if you blow up when he misbehaves and seethe with resentment because he causes so many problems—a good place to start is getting your own emotions under control.

The first step is to realize that your child doesn't make you angry: *you make yourself angry;* that is, you create your own anger by how you think about the child's behavior. When something unpleasant happens—your child throws a tantrum at a family get-together, for example—what you say to yourself about the situation will affect how you respond emotionally. If you tell yourself, "I can't stand this. How dare he embarrass me in front of all these people!" you'll be adding anger and emotional upset to an already-trying situation. If, on the other hand, you tell yourself, "This is a pain, but I'd better do what I can to defuse the situation right now," you avoid working yourself into a rage and making a bad situation even worse.

It's not easy to change the things we say to ourselves, because our ways of thinking are habits, made almost automatic by years of practice. But it can be done! You *can* change the way you respond to your child and, in doing so, you can spare yourself and your child a lot of unnecessary emotional turmoil. If you persist in your efforts, you can avoid the vicious cycle of anger, which is so destructive to your relationship with your child and which leaves you feeling so ashamed and guilty. You'll also be setting a wonderful example for your child—and we know that children learn much more from our examples than from our words.

It might help you "rethink" your responses if you remind yourself that your child is not misbehaving deliberately just to make your life miserable. Remember that children, like the rest of us, want acceptance and approval and, when they don't measure up, it's likely that it is because they *cannot,* not that they *will not.* It may help you to remain calm in difficult situations if you remind yourself that your child is just following his own "hunter-warrior" pattern and that little hunters and warriors have difficulty adapting to our world of tight schedules, breakable knick-knacks, and a million nitpicky rules.

It helps, too, to identify the *real* source of your anger, since anger often occurs in response to fear or disappointment. Certainly, ADHD children give their parents cause for disappointment and anxiety, but covering these feelings with anger won't make these feelings go away. In fact, anger just gets in the way of your ability to engage in good problem-solving. Next time you find yourself becoming angry with your ADHD child, stop and ask yourself if your anger stems from anxiety or disappointment. This helps you focus your thinking and zero in on the real source of the problem.

Getting Help for Yourself. Perhaps the self-talk strategy outlined above reminded you of cognitive therapy, discussed in Chapter 6. And that, in fact, is what it is. As noted above, changing the way you think about things is not an easy task. It's particularly difficult if you are an intense, impulsive person prone to act before you think. If you find that "talking to yourself" doesn't seem to get you anywhere, it might be helpful to spend a few sessions with a professional to get you going in the right direction.

Get professional help, too, if you fly off the handle in other situations and often feel completely overwhelmed and unable to cope. Chronic anger and irritability are common symptoms of depression. Low tolerance for stress can also signal depression, or it could be a symptom of adult ADHD. As the parent of an ADHD child, you are at high risk for both. Get treatment if you need it—for your child's sake as well as your own.

Finally, join a support group, such as CH.A.D.D. or ADDA. If none exist in your area, start one.* These groups provide emotional and social support in an atmosphere of "we're-all-in-this-together," so they can do more than even the most experienced professional to decrease a beleaguered parent's sense of isolation. Support groups are also a source of valuable information: local experts serve as speakers at monthly CH.A.D.D. meetings, for example, and newsletters are a good way to keep abreast of the latest scientific developments in the field. Some chapters maintain lending libraries and lists of local professionals who are particularly knowledgeable about ADHD. Because other parents in the group have coped with the ups and downs of life with an ADHD child, you can benefit from their fund of practical knowledge and hands-on expertise (see below).

Keeping Your Child Together

Medication and behavior-management programs can be of enormous benefit, but they are not surefire cures for all the difficulties that beset a child with ADHD. Medication, for example, doesn't help in the early morning or late night hours when it isn't in effect. How can you cope during these times? What can you do to help your disorganized little

---

* Contact the national headquarters of CH.A.D.D. and ADDA (see Appendix B) for the location of a group near you or for information about starting a group if none currently exists. Check with your child's school guidance counselor, too, for help in locating parents who might be interested in joining with you to start a support group. You could probably even use school facilities to hold meetings.

whirlwind or space cadet get himself in some semblance of order? What can you do to boost the flagging self-esteem of an ADHD youngster?

I've gleaned the following tips by asking parents what advice they would give other parents of ADHD children. What follows is a distillation of the best suggestions from parents who have grappled with the same problems you face daily.

Help Your Child Organize Himself. Because ADHD children are so scattered, they need all the help they can get to keep themselves and their belongings in order.

■ Clear out the clutter in your child's room. The more furniture, toys, and books in the room, the harder it is to clean. It's harder, too, to find the things your child needs when he needs them. Wardrobes should also be simplified: many children have two or three favorite outfits that they wear constantly. Instead of scrambling frantically to wash the same shirt three times a week or dealing with wails of dismay when it's in the laundry, buy duplicates of favorite items. (This also makes it easier for your child to put together an outfit that doesn't require you to wear blinders when you're in the same room with him.)

■ Spell out all expectations. Put a chart on the bathroom door to remind him that he needs to brush his teeth every morning and that taking a shower means using soap as well as shampoo. You'll still have to check on him, but the charts will help a lot.

Set Priorities and Keep Things in Perspective. Decide what's important and what doesn't really matter. Then act accordingly.

■ High-achieving families must be careful to avoid an overemphasis on grades and academic achievement. Success in school is important, but it isn't as important as the child's self-esteem and a close relationship with his parents. If you and your child are constantly at war over his schoolwork, ask yourself if it's really worth throwing away your precious time with your child in this fashion. As Dr. Russell Barkley pointedly asks, is it worth the loss of your relationship with your child?[153]

■ Holidays can be difficult for ADHD children because they respond to the excitement around them and spiral out of control. Take a long, hard look at what is important to you about the holidays and then pare things down. If you wear yourself out with cooking, baking, decorating, and shopping, you won't have any patience left to deal with your ADHD child.

■ If you and your child seem to lock horns over every little thing, stand back and consider what's really important in terms of the child's health, safety, and welfare. Hold your ground on those issues but be prepared to give ground on little things, like whether or not he folds his laundry before he puts it away: you might value a tidy drawer with all underwear neatly folded, but your child probably couldn't care less. Remember, in all of recorded history, there is not a single known case of death due to wearing unfolded underwear.

Recognize and Respect Your Child's Limits. Because ADHD is an invisible handicap, parents often forget that their child may have difficulty with tasks and responsibilities that others their age have mastered. If you find yourself constantly frustrated and disappointed with your ADHD child, it may be a red flag that you are overestimating his abilities and setting yourself up for disappointment.

■ Think ahead in situations in which your child might have particular problems and don't put him in a position of assured failure. If Aunt Ethel has dozens of knickknacks all over the house and won't put them out of reach when you visit, *don't visit.* If birthday parties and large family gatherings bring out the worst in your child, plan to arrive late and leave early. In between, watch for signs that the child is becoming overstimulated and be prepared to remove him before trouble starts.

■ Make your expectations fit the child, not the other way around. Stick with the reality of what your child can do and work from there. For example, even if other children his age can dress themselves in the morning, your child may not be able to do this without help. Either recognize this and adjust your morning schedule so you can provide this help or be prepared for a nasty scene every morning: the choice is yours.

Boost Your Child's Self-Esteem. The term self-esteem seems on the way to becoming another buzzword in the lexicon of American parents. It's too bad, because ADHD youngsters need all the help they can get in this department.

■ Remember to compliment your child as often as you can. This is especially important for ADHD children, because they usually receive so many negative comments and so few compliments. Praise doesn't have to be lavish: a simple "thanks" and a smile or a hug can be more powerful than you know. (P.S. This goes a long way with spouses too!)

▪ Find and foster any activity in which your child excels, such as sports, music, or art. Because of their energy and intensity, many ADHD youngsters have a flair for the dramatic arts and find satisfaction and success in little theater groups and acting classes. Get the child involved in youth activities at your church or synagogue, where supportive people will express appreciation for the child's contributions.

▪ Get your child a pet. Pets offer unconditional love and they don't criticize children for their shortcomings. However, don't be so naïve as to assume that your ADHD child will actually assume responsibility for the pet's care, in spite of all promises to the contrary: every day, as I look out my window, I see my neighbors walking the dogs their children promised to walk.

And *don't* get pets for very young, very impulsive ADHD children, because someone, either child or pet, is bound to get hurt. I recall an adorable little perpetual-motion machine in the form of a five-year-old who informed me that the family no longer had their dog because, he explained indignantly, "He attacked me!" "He attacked you?" I repeated. "Yeah. I bit him in the nose and he attacked me."*

Keeping Your Marriage Together

Because the stress involved in raising a youngster with ADHD can put so much pressure on a marriage, your relationship with your spouse may need special attention. If you think you don't have time to devote to your marriage, spend a few minutes thinking about how you would fare as a divorced parent, raising your ADHD child alone.

Get Out and About. As a clinical psychologist, I've learned to expect blank stares when I ask parents of ADHD children, "How long has it been since the two of you spent a weekend—or even an evening—without the kids?" Even when parents do spend time alone together, too

---

* Labrador Retrievers and Golden Retrievers tend to be more patient with children than many other breeds and are often a good choice for ADHD children. Avoid the more nervous, high-strung breeds such as Schnauzers and Dalmations if you have an impulsive ADHD youngster.

often this precious time is taken up with discussing the ADHD child and his problems.

If your preoccupation with your child's problems colors your time together as a couple, plan activities that force your attention away from your child's problems to the activity at hand. The more engrossing the activity, the better: it's hard to worry about problems at home when you're piloting a raft through white water or trying to keep your balance at a skating rink or cheering for the home team at a ball game. Sign up for tennis lessons together. Go to a play or a movie. Visit friends who have no children: if you are tempted to go on and on about your child's difficulties, their glazed looks will force a quick change of topic.

Respect Each Other's Style. As noted earlier, ADHD children often behave better for Dad than for Mom. This can be maddening for a mother, particularly if her husband assumes that this is due to his superior parenting skills and insists that his wife would get good results if she would just adopt his parenting style.

With these fathers, I point out that most children behave better for their fathers than for their mothers. Thousands of years of evolution have shaped men and women to assume very different roles as parents. Women are the nurturers and the caregivers, the ones who feed, soothe, cuddle and generally minister to the needs of their young. On the other hand, nature seems to have intended that males be the representatives of law and order: "I'm in charge here and you'd better respect that, or else!"*

From this perspective, it's understandable that mothers and fathers have very different parenting styles. It's not surprising, either, that tactics that work well for one do not work well for the other and that neither parent can easily assume the style that comes so naturally to the other. If we observe mothers interacting with their children, we see that they are much less likely than fathers to jump in with harsh corrections and threats of punishment. Instead, they are more likely to use strategies such as reasoning, negotiation, and distraction.

The problem is that these time-honored parenting strategies don't work very well with ADHD children. Why not? Let's take a close look.

---

* If this strikes you as hard to believe, pay a visit to the local zoo and observe the bears, the tigers, and the lions. Whose tail is being used in a game of tug-of-war? Whose ears are being mauled by the cubs? You can bet it's not Papa Bear's!

▪ **Reasoning.** Where will reasoning get you with an ADHD child? As psychologist Tom Phelan[154] humorously but accurately reminds us, children are not little adults; they are not reasonable creatures who will alter their behavior when given a sensible reason for doing so. They will not, for example, say "Oh, yes, I didn't realize that" when you tell them a cookie ten minutes before dinner will spoil their appetite for healthier food. Nor will they respond "Gosh, you're right" when you point out that they are old enough to pick up after themselves, carry their plates to the kitchen, or make their own beds.

Instead, they will interpret your reason simply as your opening argument and will happily respond in kind, giving you a thousand and one "reasons" why your reason is all wet. As anyone who has ever lived with an ADHD child knows, these youngsters are born litigators who love a debate and would gladly argue with a possum. If you give them an opening argument, they'll take it and run with it to the point of exhaustion. Unfortunately, you'll become exhausted long before they will.

▪ **Negotiation.** Negotiation seldom works with ADHD youngsters, for the reason cited above. Any offer to negotiate is perceived as the opening move in a game of "the-sky-is-the-limit."

> PARENT: If you finish your homework by six o'clock, you can watch an hour of television before bed.
>
> CHILD: No, if I finish my homework by six o'clock, you have to buy me three new video games, let me stay up till midnight, and let me have ten kids for a sleepover on Friday night.

If you negotiate with an ADHD child, be sure that you hold the winning cards. Otherwise, be prepared for a lengthy debate that will get you nowhere. Often, a simple declarative statement such as "This is not a choice" is an effective way to end the conversation.

▪ **Distraction.** A toddler who is headed toward Aunt Mildred's Ming vase can often be diverted by mother's keys or a toy dangled in an inviting manner. An older child can be coaxed away from interfering with a sibling's activity by a parent's offer to play a game, bake some cookies, or go for a walk.

Although this time-honored strategy works with some children, it's usually doomed to fail with ADHD children because, while ADHD children have the attention span of a gnat for things like homework, they have tunnel vision concerning things they themselves want to do. Then, nothing short of a nuclear attack can divert them from their objective.

In fact, when distraction fails as a first line of intervention so that the parent must take sterner measures and reprimand the child ("No. Stop that!"), children often respond with fussing and tantrums.[155] Since the tantrums of an ADHD child can approach the spectacular, parents of ADHD children would be better advised to respond first to any unacceptable behavior, no matter how minor, with a quick "No." Then *follow* the reprimand with distraction ("You can have this instead").

It's easy to see, then, that the tactics most mothers employ with their children are ineffective with ADHD children. However, when mothers try to implement the strategies that work well for fathers, that, too, can backfire because ADHD children often respond with redoubled efforts, and ugly power struggles can result. Therefore, rather than trying to mimic a style that works for Dad, mothers would do better to adopt a more "gender neutral" approach, such as Tom Phelan's "1-2-3: Magic" method, described in Chapter 6.

But what about consistency? Haven't we heard a million times that ADHD children in particular need consistency? If we are talking about prompt and consistent consequences for misbehavior, the answer is yes. In fact, researchers have found that if parents respond permissively to misbehavior or confuse the child by sometimes permitting or rewarding the behavior and at other times by reprimanding the child, the results are high rates of misbehavior and lots of tantrums.[156] If consistency means that one parent supports the decision of the other, rather than undercutting the other parent, the answer is also yes.

On the other hand, consistency doesn't mean that parents must be carbon copies of each other in terms of the behaviors they will not tolerate or the consequences they impose. If Dad doesn't mind playing short-order cook and producing a different meal for each child when Mom's working late, she shouldn't insist that Dad impose her rule of "Eat what is in front of you" in her absence. And if Dad can't stand fussing and teasing while he's trying to watch the news, he's within his rights to send noisy little squabblers to their rooms so he can have peace, even if Mom doesn't find their behavior so trying.

Helping Siblings Cope

Anyone who believes that brothers and sisters should get along in perfect harmony is obviously an only child! In the real world, siblings are pitted from the start in an intense and never-ending competition to be first and best in the eyes of their parents.

In fact, studies show that there is actually a surprising amount of violence between siblings in average American families.[157] In families in which there are one or more members with ADHD, it's likely that the rates are even higher, because active, bouncy ADHD children can be so annoying to their siblings. And when they in turn are annoyed with a brother or sister, their impulsivity and poor frustration tolerance make it likely that physical retaliation will be involved.

Sibling battles, however normal, are aggravating to parents, and they probably don't do much good for the kids themselves either. If your house resembles a war zone, what can you do to bring about some degree of peace among your children?

■ As the authority figures in the family, you must protect the property rights and physical security of all members of the family. If locks are needed to ensure privacy and protect property, use them. If physical fights are common between siblings who are unevenly matched in terms of size and strength, the rule must be crystal clear: no physical contact of any sort, at any time—period. Enforce the rule swiftly and firmly. Don't ask who started it: "He hit me first" does not excuse hitting back.

■ What about name-calling? If you can ignore it, fine. If it makes you crazy to hear your children address each other as "Poop-head" and "Stupid-butt," try this little tactic next time there's a war of the words.

Tell the children that you understand their need to express their angry feelings. Take them into a remote part of the house (the basement or garage will work nicely), give them a tape recorder, and instruct them to spend exactly thirty minutes calling each other names. Tell them that you will listen to the tape on your way to work the next day and that if there are any blank spots on the tape, they will have to do the entire exercise again.

Once around with this routine and you'll find that all you have to do the next time name-calling begins is hold up your tape recorder and inquire sweetly, "Do we need a recording session?"

■ Don't fall into the "it's-not-fair" trap. This problem is especially pronounced in families with an ADHD child. You can't resolve the problem by arguing about whether the complaints are legitimate or even by trying to make things fair and equal for all children in the family. That's not what it's all about. Instead, as Adele Faber and Elaine Mazlish suggest in their wonderful book, *Siblings Without Rivalry,*★ recognize the child's complaint for what it really is: a bid for reassurance that he is special and beloved. If you recognize this—if you listen carefully to the child's complaint and empathize with his feelings—you'll often find that the problem resolves itself without further intervention from you.

To learn more about this sensible approach to problems of sibling rivalry, read the book. It's even endorsed by Ann Landers!

■ Stress cooperation instead of competition. This, of course, falls into the easier-said-than-done category, since siblings are naturally so competitive. You can, however, glean some very good tips from Faber and Mazlish's book, cited above.

You can also encourage cooperation by rewarding group performance rather than individual performance. For example, instead of saying "Let's see who can be the first one ready for bed," you might say "If everyone is ready for bed by eight, we can make some popcorn." Be careful, though, that this doesn't backfire and result in the successful children exploding in fury at the child whose lack of success results in a lost treat for all. To forestall this, set goals that all children in the family can meet and explain to the children that they are more assured of success if they work as a team.

Finally, reward loving, cooperative behavior when you see it. You'll get a lot more mileage out of "I love to see you being so helpful to each other" than from criticizing or punishing uncooperative behavior—and it's so much more pleasant for all concerned. Reward "positive tattling" too. Wouldn't you like to hear "Mommy, Johnny shared his candy with me" rather than "Mommy, Johnny took the ball away from me?" If so, teach this behavior and reward it when it occurs.

■ Keep your expectations reasonable. Don't expect your other chil-

★ New York: Avon Books, 1988.

dren to tolerate annoying behavior from their ADHD sibling just because "he has a problem." The explanation "He can't help it" doesn't make much sense to children, especially young children. Children firmly believe that all acts are intentional: the bottom line to them is "He did it—period."

Just as you can help your ADHD child learn to distinguish intentionally hostile acts from accidents, as we discussed earlier, you can also help your other children understand that the ADHD child can't easily foresee the consequences of his own actions. The critical point, however, is to acknowledge that the child who was erred against has a right to be upset and disgruntled. "Kerry was just goofing around. I don't think she really meant to make you so angry, but I can see that it ticked you off." Again, refer to *Siblings Without Rivalry* for sensitive ways in which to listen to, and defuse, a child's anger.

Nontraditional Families and ADHD Children

So far we've talked about the kinds of problems ADHD children and their family members experience when the ADHD child lives in an intact family with his biological parents and siblings. But what about ADHD children in other kinds of family settings—adoptive families, for example, or single-parent families? Many ADHD children live in such nontraditional families and, in many ways, their difficulties are even more complex than those of ADHD children raised in an intact family with biological parents. So complex is their situation, in fact, that we can do little more here than highlight some of the issues and offer some broad recommendations.

Adopted Children with ADHD

There is growing awareness that many adopted youngsters, especially those who are adopted at an older age or adopted from developing countries, are at very high risk for ADHD.[158] Much of the risk can be attributed to genetic factors; some perhaps results from poor prenatal care and/or neglect or abuse prior to adoption.

If you are the parent of an adopted child with ADHD, you—like your child—face something of a "double whammy": not only must you both contend with the fact of ADHD; you also have to deal with all the issues surrounding the fact of the adoption itself. Adopted children, for example, have to grapple with the fact that they were relinquished by their birth parents, an act that may leave them with a nagging sense of not having been "good enough" to have been kept. When the adopted child also struggles with ADHD, problems with self-esteem are likely to occur.

Other problems, too, face the adopted ADHD child:

- Adopted children often see themselves as different from children who have "real" parents. This sense of being different may be magnified when the adopted child has to take medication, go to a psychiatrist, and is in other ways set apart by virtue of ADHD.

- To adopted children, the expectations of their parents seem high and many feel incapable of living up to these expectations. For adopted children with ADHD, it may seem that it would be easier to scale Mount Everest barefoot than to live up to the expectations of their adoptive parents.

- Identity conflicts in adolescence can be particularly painful and confusing for adopted ADHD youngsters. To "You don't understand me" is added "You *would* if you were my real parents." At the same time, the communication problems common between parents and teenagers are often increased by the fact that adoptive parents are often several years older than the parents of the child's friends and classmates.

Implications for Parents. As an adoptive parent of an ADHD youngster, you might benefit from suggestions offered by other parents in the same boat. These suggestions were garnered in a survey of more than three hundred families of adopted ADHD children conducted by Robin Allen, director of the Barker Foundation in Cabin John, Maryland.[159]

- Don't try to go it alone. Join a support group for parents of ADHD children. If you're lucky enough to live in an area where there are special support groups for adoptive parents of ADHD children, join and become an active member. If not, consider starting such a group yourself.

- Stay "in sync" with your child by encouraging open talk about feelings and thoughts surrounding adoption and ADHD. Don't be too quick to jump in with reassuring platitudes about loving the child just the way he or she is. Instead, just listen to your child's concerns; sometimes, just feeling like they've been heard is enough to defuse strong or overwhelming emotions.

And, as the adoptive parent of one of my ADHD patients noted, "When things get bad, I remind myself that this is truly my opportunity to make a difference in a life."

ADHD Children in Divorced Families

As difficult as it is to raise an ADHD child in an intact family, it's harder to do so alone, as a single parent. Like the parent of an adopted child with ADHD, you're faced with a double layer of difficulty—your child's problems and the problems you have with your former spouse.

Your child, too, must deal with a dual set of problems because, even if you and your former spouse have parted amicably, separation and divorce bring their own problems and losses for children. These losses go beyond the obvious loss of a parent to include loss of a familiar home, school, neighborhood, and friends. Often, too, there is a drop in the standard of living, since resources that were adequate for one family now must be stretched to cover two families.

For children of divorce, the most painful of all losses occurs when the noncustodial parent is irregular with visits. Unfortunately, since biological parents of ADHD children are so often ADHD themselves, many an ADHD child finds himself wondering when or if his noncustodial parent will arrive for a promised visit.

Unfortunately, too, with ADHD children there are unique opportunities for warring parents to put their ADHD child squarely in the middle of their battles. Sometimes battles center around obtaining appropriate treatment for the child: often, for example, one parent adamantly denies that the child has ADHD, arguing that there is nothing wrong with the child or that any problems the child manifests stem from the divorce or from the poor parenting skills of the other parent.

This parent usually can be counted on to do all in his or her power to sabotage treatment, including actively discouraging the child from taking medication. This, of course, puts the child in an impossible position, particularly if the child is eager to maintain a close relationship with the dissenting parent.

Warring parents also use problems that crop up when the child is in transition from one parent's home to another as "proof" that the other parent is insensitive to the child's needs and is, therefore, an unfit parent. What these parents fail to realize, however, is that transition times are tough on all children of divorce, especially those whose parents have not resolved their own problems. When the child must cross the equivalent of a mine field between battling parents, the stress takes a heavy toll. And since ADHD children tend to become more active, disorganized, and difficult under stress, nasty and upsetting scenes are inevitable.

Implications for Parents. Even parents who disagree about everything else concerning their ADHD child will usually acknowledge that divorce is hard on children and that many children of divorce can benefit from counseling. Certainly, the need for this kind of intervention is particularly pronounced with ADHD children, who already have more than their fair share of baggage. A competent professional can not only help the child work through the emotional turmoil associated with a divorce, he or she can also help by providing specific advice and recommendations to help you help your child through all the changes a divorce brings.

But not even the most competent professional can help if you and your former spouse remain locked in mortal combat. If this is the case, do whatever it takes to help both of you—or at least one of you—put aside your corrosive anger. Go through mediation with your former spouse and be prepared to give some ground for the sake of your child. Go into individual therapy. Talk with your priest, minister, or rabbi. Pray, meditate, take up yoga. The point is that as long as you and your child's other parent are at war, your child will experience emotional pain.

For other suggestions on helping your ADHD child—or any child—survive the wrenching experience of divorce, I recommend Dr. Elissa Benedek's book, *How to Help Your Child Overcome Your Divorce.**

---

* Washington, D.C.: American Psychiatric Press, 1995.

When a Parent Has ADHD

Since ADHD has a strong hereditary component, it's a good bet that where you find a child with ADHD, you will also find at least one parent with it as well. It's one thing, however, to cope with impulsive, scattered, volatile behavior in a ten-year-old and something else again to cope with the same behaviors in your marriage partner.

> "The experts can tell you a lot about what to do for a child who has ADHD. But what if your husband has it too? My husband is a wonderful guy and I love him dearly, but it's like having another child in the house. He can't remember anything I ask him to do, whether it's 'Pick up milk on your way home' or even 'Pick up the kids on your way home.' Last week, my daughter called in a panic because she'd been waiting for her dad to pick her up after practice and he never showed up.
>
> "I keep the checkbook and pay our bills because he's lost when it comes to managing money. I don't mind that, but I can't even ask him to put the bills in the mail—they just sit in his truck, gathering dust, until I get a call from the landlord about the rent check that's overdue."

The Problems

The havoc that the presence of an ADHD adult can wreak in a family and the toll it can take on a spouse have been described in detail in several books on adult ADHD.[160,161,162] What kinds of problems do these writers describe?

Narcissism. According to these authors and others, one of the most common problems is that ADHD adults often come across as selfish and self-absorbed—"narcissistic," in psychiatric jargon. Certainly, many of their behavior patterns call to mind the god Narcissus, who was so enamored of his own image in a reflecting pool that he fell in and drowned. ADHD adults don't seem to listen to other people; they interrupt with their own concerns and go off on their own tangents. They forget things that are important to those around them, like birthdays and anniversaries.

They make lavish, heartfelt promises but fail to follow through, leaving others disappointed and angry.

Volatile Moods. As Dr. Paul Wender, an authority on adult ADHD notes, adults with ADHD often have rapid mood shifts.[163] They also blow up over little annoyances and, although they may calm down quickly, people around them often remain shaken and upset for hours. Many explosive ADHD adults don't realize how frightening their outbursts are to others until it's too late and valued relationships are damaged beyond repair.

Poor Conflict Resolution Skills. In a troubled marriage, it's common for spouses to dredge up past wrongs and drag them into every argument. This pattern, sometimes known as "garbage collecting" or, as Hallowell and Ratey term it, "kitchen sinking," virtually ensures that the dispute at hand will be lost under the weight of accumulated grievances, rather than being resolved.

Unfortunately, this practice is particularly likely to derail attempts to resolve conflict when an ADHD person is involved because of the distractibility associated with ADHD.

Communication Problems. Miscommunication can be a serious problem in marriages in which a partner has ADHD because receptive and expressive language disorders often go hand in hand with ADHD, as we discussed in Chapter 2. The real-life example below illustrates how easily communication can become hopelessly snarled.

Carole and Ann were chatting over coffee when their friend Dave, an adult with ADHD, joined them. The conversation turned to the subject of dogs, and Carole mentioned that she'd recently acquired a beagle.

ANN: Oh, they are such cute dogs. I bet you just love him.

CAROLE: He is cute, but he's got a mind of his own. He's going to be a challenge to train.

DAVE: Well, how did you train your other dogs? That should work for him, too, if it worked for the others.

CAROLE: *(Puzzled)* Huh? What "other dogs"? I don't know what you mean.

DAVE: Well, Ann said "dogs," so I thought you had a couple of them. Don't you?

When this kind of problem with receptive language is compounded by the fact that people with ADHD are intense and tend to express themselves in exaggerated fashion ("I'll just kill myself if I can't get this done" versus "Gee, I really want to finish this"), it's easy to see how serious communication problems can result.

Remember, too, that men and women have different communication styles—so different, in fact, that they might as well be from different planets, as the title of *Men Are from Mars, Women Are from Venus** suggests.

Scientists who study linguistics, such as Dr. Deborah Tannen at Georgetown University, tell us that men and women use language very differently.[164] They even listen differently: men signal attention to the speaker by listening quietly, while women use gestures and comments such as "um hm" and "yeah" to indicate that they are listening. Since men and women actually use different parts of their brains when speaking, these differences in style are understandable. However, they are a chronic source of misunderstanding between the sexes.

When we add up all of the factors that complicate communication in a marriage in which one partner has ADHD, it's not surprising that misunderstandings commonly occur. On the contrary: it's amazing that anything ever gets communicated at all.

Comorbid Psychiatric Problems. Just as children with ADHD often have coexisting psychiatric problems that go undetected, so, too, do ADHD adults. In terms of relationship problems, chief among these conditions is depression. In fact, experts believe that few disorders have as much impact on interpersonal relations as depression does.

In marriages in which one spouse suffers from depression, for example, interactions between the partners are considerably more negative and hostile than in marriages in which neither partner is depressed.[165] Little constructive problem-solving takes place in these couples, so the partners become caught in a destructive cycle of frustration, withdrawal, and mistrust.[166]

Other comorbid problems also affect the intimate relationships of ADHD adults. Certainly, alcoholism is high on the list of problems that contribute to marital battles. Alcoholism and drug abuse also greatly in-

* New York: HarperCollins, 1992.

crease the risk of violence and abuse, problems that may be more common in families with an ADHD member than in other families.

Steps Toward Resolution

If you recognize your marriage in the preceding sections, what can you do to change things? Maybe you've already tried marital counseling and found it to be of little help. Certainly, you've tried talking, persuading, nagging—even threatening divorce. What else can you do?

If marriage counseling failed in the past, it might be because ADHD or coexisting problems were not taken into consideration. Talk therapy can be very helpful under some circumstances, as discussed in Chapter 6. But talk therapy can't curb the impulsivity, volatility, and other ADHD-associated problems that complicate and confound intimate relationships.

The first step, then, is to obtain a good evaluation from a professional who is knowledgeable about adult ADHD. Professionals with this kind of expertise aren't like buses that come along every fifteen minutes, so you may have to shop around before you find one who has the skills to address your needs. Your child's psychologist or psychiatrist might be able to help with a referral or even provide an evaluation. If not, ask for referrals from members of your support group.

Depending on the recommendations of the professional you consult, you might be given a prescription for medication. Again, we find that men and women react very differently to such a recommendation. Women are usually eager to access the benefits that medication offers, while men are more apt to see medication as an artificial aid or crutch and, therefore, a sign of weakness. I point out that eyeglasses are also artificial aids, as are toothpaste, soap, and deodorant. Could we do without them? Certainly. But I would rather not, would you?

Do a little work on your own too. Read as much as you can about adult ADHD to gain insight into the problems associated with ADHD and to gather ideas for bringing about change. Talk with other ADHD adults or with a "coach" to find out what has worked for others. Go to meetings and conferences on ADHD: you'll learn a lot and you'll have a good time too.

Finally, try to keep your sense of humor alive. You—and your marriage—will live much longer if you do.

CHAPTER 9

SCHOOL DAYS, SCHOOL DAZE

Overview: Then and Now

Then: Federal laws guaranteeing handicapped children an appropriate education were in place a decade ago. However, since ADHD children were not specifically named in federal legislation, many were denied the accommodations and services they needed to function well in school.

Parents and teachers were often on opposing sides in an ugly battle. Teachers blamed parents for the unacceptable behavior of their ADHD children, while parents accused teachers of being insensitive to the legitimate needs of the child—needs that went unmet as the battle raged.

Now: Great strides have been made in a decade. Parents of ADHD children across the country breathed a huge sigh of relief when a memo from the U.S. Department of Education specifically stated that ADHD children were potentially eligible for special education services under two separate federal laws.

Although there are still some diehards who resist what they see as "coddling" children with ADHD, teachers today are generally much better informed about the needs of ADHD children and how to meet these needs in the classroom. In many school systems, classroom teachers now work with resource teachers and guidance counselors to put special accommodations in place for ADHD children even before these children are formally diagnosed and a written plan of action is developed.

Round Pegs, Square Holes

Many ADHD children do reasonably well until they enter school. There, faced with the academic and social demands of the classroom, they encounter failure and frustration as they try to fit into a setting for which Mother Nature clearly did not design them.

Some ADHD children, especially those who are aggressive toward peers and disobedient and defiant toward adults, are identified in preschool. As discussed earlier, these youngsters are particularly likely to have comorbid problems in addition to rather severe ADHD.

Many sociable, good-natured ADHD youngsters do not begin to falter until they encounter the demands of elementary school—demands to remain seated and attentive during teacher presentations; to work independently for sustained periods of time; and to change activities quickly when the schedule dictates.

Some ADHD youngsters—usually those who are quite bright and personable—make it to middle school or high school before they crash and burn. Some have coasted on their intelligence; others have relied on collaboration between a well-organized mother and understanding teachers to get them through the elementary-school years.

In middle school and high school, however, teachers focus on the curriculum rather than on the individual child. And even the most organized parent cannot maintain close contact with five or six teachers. Faced with reduced teacher support, multiple classes, and an increased workload, many of these youngsters "hit the wall" and come to professional attention for the first time.

Finding a Better Fit

Traditional classrooms are not very user-friendly to active, impulsive ADHD children who love change, excitement, and novelty. In classrooms where children must remain seated while doing assigned work or listening to the teacher present a lesson, ADHD children are likely to daydream, fidget, squirm, make strange noises, move around a lot, and generally annoy those around them. On the other hand, ADHD children are much less likely to stand out from their classmates in classrooms where children are allowed to select activities and work at their own pace.

Alternatives to Public School. This may explain why some ADHD children who do well in a Montessori program fall apart in more traditional educational settings. If Montessori programs are available into the elementary school years, or if other nontraditional schools that focus on the "whole child" (e.g., the Waldorf schools) are available, parents often ask if the child should remain in such a school as long as possible. I am inclined to think so. If problems arise when the child eventually transfers to a more traditional school, we can deal with them at that time (although I've found that most youngsters make the transition quite smoothly): in the interim, as long as the child is happy and successful, leave well enough alone!

Some parents take the opposite tack: hoping that a more challenging academic program will infuse motivation into a bright but underachieving ADHD student, they enroll the child in honors courses or programs for gifted children. Sometimes this works well: the child's imagination is fired by a brilliant teacher or an exciting hands-on program. More often, however, a child whose performance is lackluster in regular classes will continue to perform below par in a more advanced program.

Still other parents assume that a private school, with smaller classrooms and more individual attention, might be a better environment for an ADHD child. Some private schools, especially those that specialize in working with learning-disabled children, can meet the needs of ADHD children. In general, however, private schools lack the resources and the range of expertise available in the public school system. Further, some academically competitive private schools are unwilling to provide accommodations for children with special needs.

Before you enroll your child in a private school—indeed, before you make any decisions about educational placement—it's a good idea to consult an educational placement specialist. These professionals, who usually have a background in education or child psychology, have first-hand knowledge about a broad range of programs and services in both private and public schools in the area and are experts at matching children with schools and programs most likely to foster success.

In any school, it's the teacher who sets the tone and style in the classroom. The teacher's tolerance level and skill in working with children who march to a different drum are critical factors in how well the ADHD child fares in her classroom. The teacher's role vis-à-vis children with ADHD is discussed in the next section.

Guidelines for Teachers

The Teacher-Child Relationship

Teachers who attend workshops on ADHD hope to learn specific tactics to help them deal with the ADHD youngsters in their classrooms. Some are dismayed to learn that while there are many things teachers can do to help their ADHD students, there are no tricks, no quick fixes, and no one-size-fits-all treatment strategies.

Instead, the most effective teachers of ADHD children understand that their relationship with the child is the single most powerful agent of change available to them. When the relationship works—when there is mutual respect and understanding between teacher and child—the ADHD child can soar to wonderful heights. Unfortunately, the reverse is true as well: when the fit between child and teacher is poor, the ADHD child is in for a miserable year and so is everyone else around him.

"Greg had a miserable year in fourth grade. Every morning, it was a fight to get him out of bed and ready for school. Every day it was some excuse: 'I'm too tired.' 'My head aches.' 'My stomach hurts.' We got so worried that we took him to his pediatrician for a checkup but he couldn't find a thing wrong with him.

"This year, he's a different child. He rushes to school every morning to take care of the classroom pets before school starts. That's his special job because Mrs. Bailey knows how much he loves animals. He's so proud that Mrs. Bailey trusts him with this job: he'd rather die than let her down. And it's really made a difference in his schoolwork too. Mrs. Bailey told him that she didn't want to overburden him—that if he couldn't keep up with his work and still care for the animals, she'd see about finding someone else who could help with the animals. That was all he needed to hear! He hasn't missed an assignment since then."

But what if your child isn't in Mrs. Bailey's class? What if he's in a class with a teacher who doesn't seem to understand him at all? When this happens, try to work things out quickly and amicably. Request a meeting with the teacher and ask to have the guidance counselor and principal included. Don't come in with guns blazing. Instead, be honest in discussing your child's shortcomings. Acknowledge the fact that your child's behavior can be very trying in the classroom, if that is indeed the case.

If the teacher and others in the school seem receptive, offer to provide educational materials (the *CH.A.D.D. Educators Manual* and *The ADD Hyperactivity Handbook for Schools* are good choices: see Resources at the end of this chapter). You might also contact your local CH.A.D.D. chapter to see if someone can provide a free or low-cost inservice program for all of the teachers in your child's school.

The View from the Teacher's Desk. Of course, it's easy to understand how an ADHD child can antagonize his teachers. In a class of twenty-five children, a child who makes strange noises, interrupts constantly, bugs his neighbors, and demands help with the simplest of tasks can make even a dedicated teacher seriously consider a career change. Consider the following classroom observations made by the guidance counselor of a nine-year-old boy with ADHD.

9:55   Mrs. Mather is explaining a math problem to the class. Eric is playing with something in his desk. Mrs. Mather asks, "Eric, are you paying attention?" Eric says, "What?"

10:00   Eric is rolling a pencil around on his desk. Mrs. Mather calls Eric and two other children to sign up for science projects. Eric goes to the bulletin board and signs up.

10:05   The other children return to their seats. Eric walks over to another boy and asks if he has signed up yet. He returns to his desk after poking another child in the arm in passing.

10:10   Eric is standing next to his desk. Mrs. Mather comes over and tells him to get back to work. Eric says, "I *am* working. I don't know how to do these problems" (the problems Mrs. Mather has just explained to the class). Mrs. Mather goes over a problem with him, checks the ones he has done, and tells him to redo a couple of them. She leaves. He looks around the room.

10:15   Eric calls out, "Mrs. Mather!" She responds, "I asked you to redo those problems." Eric says, "I did. I still don't understand." Mrs. Mather points out something on his paper and he starts to work, still standing beside his desk. Now he stares at a pen and plays with it while looking around the room. He starts to hum.

10:20   As another boy walks past him, Eric pokes him and giggles. The other boy looks annoyed and says, "Quit it, Eric." Eric laughs and makes a face.

10:30   Mrs. Mather tells the class to take out their spelling folders. Eric looks in his backpack while Mrs. Mather waits, then asks him, "Do you have your spelling folder?" Eric appears agitated and yells, "I can't find it!" Mrs. Mather comes over to help.

A youngster like Eric can make every day a teacher's day from hell. On a teacher's stress meter, he's a "ten" most days—and even higher on his bad days.

The View from the Child's Desk. Teachers find it infuriating that the ADHD child never seems to see how his own behavior contributes to his difficulties. Instead, he blames others for problems that are obviously of his own making: when confronted with wrongdoing, his stock replies are "It's not fair," "It wasn't my fault," and "I didn't do anything."

But these complaints make sense when we look at things from the child's point of view. In an enlightening study[167] of how children interpret the actions of their teachers and classmates, children were given a fictional example of a child who was active, impulsive, and disruptive in the classroom. They were asked *why* they thought the child behaved the way he did, *how* their own teacher would respond to such behavior, and *why* she would respond as she did.

The interpretations given by ADHD children differed strikingly from those given by other children. Asked why the fictional child behaved as he did, non-ADHD children believed that the child was deliberately misbehaving, while ADHD children believed that the behavior was beyond the child's ability to control. Both groups predicted that their teacher would respond negatively to the disruptive behavior but, while the non-ADHD children saw the teacher as just "doing her job," ADHD children saw her reactions as stemming from *personal dislike of the disruptive child.*

As the author of this study pointed out, ADHD children don't believe that they are in control of their behavior. Thus, negative reactions from teachers and classmates seem unfair, since it is obviously unfair to punish someone for actions beyond his control. And why would a teacher punish unfairly unless she disliked the offending child?

This study helps us understand the defensive reactions of the ADHD child. From his point of view, he is not out to get the teacher: the teacher is out to get him!

How can you, as a teacher, help an ADHD child understand how his behavior affects others and why they react to him as they do? One way is to tell the child how others interpret his behavior and to explain the rationale for their own behavior toward the child.* For example:

> "When you wiggle around in your seat and make noises, it bothers the children near you. They think you do it on purpose, so sometimes they get mad at you. Maybe if you sit next to me that will help you sit and do your work."
>
> "I know you didn't mean any harm, but the rule is 'No touching others.' Poking other people makes them angry. They think you mean to hurt them. Please keep your hands in your pockets when you walk across the room. That will help you remember not to touch people."
>
> "If you make a lot of noise in the hall, it bothers children in other classes. Maybe they're taking a big test or doing something else that's important to them. Their teachers would be upset with me if I let my children disturb their children. Walk beside me and I'll help you walk quietly."

This approach conveys concern for the child. It also helps the child gain some self-awareness and prevents misunderstandings between teacher and child.

---

* Research has shown that all children—not just those with ADHD—do better when they are given a brief rationale for the rules they are expected to follow.

Providing Structure and Feedback

By definition, ADHD youngsters are scattered, forgetful, absentminded, and disorganized. They are also prone to daydream, dawdle, doodle, and engage in a thousand other off-task activities in the classroom. What can a teacher do to keep these helter-skelter children organized and on task?

The Importance of Structure and Organization. Because ADHD children can't organize themselves in time or in space, others must assume this responsibility for them long after other children have learned to organize themselves. Organizational skills can't be taught to the ADHD child on a one-shot basis, as many well-intentioned people think and as many a parent who has enrolled an ADHD youngster in an organizational-skills course has learned.

Instead, we must recognize that poor organizational skills are a hallmark of ADHD, much as muscular weakness is associated with many orthopedic conditions. And while we provide the orthopedically handicapped child with physical therapy to strengthen his weak muscles, we would never assume that after one course the child could cast aside his crutches or leap from his wheelchair and stride across the room. Rather, we would continue to provide the special support the child needed to function at his best in the classroom.

What kind of organizational support do ADHD students need? Several years ago, I had the opportunity to observe the special classroom at the National Institute of Mental Health for children who were participating in research programs there. As I noted in *Your Hyperactive Child,* this classroom was a model of organization and structure. What made this classroom special?

- **Clear rules.** It stands to reason that children are more likely to follow rules if they know exactly what the rules are. Yet, researchers tell us that even when teachers firmly believe that they have taught classroom rules, only a small number of children in the primary grades can actually state or identify the rules pertaining to their own classroom.[168] Rules should be posted, discussed in detail, and made salient by pointing out examples of students following them.

- **Precise instructions.** With ADHD youngsters, a general directive like "Line up to go to recess" would probably produce pushing, shoving, and pandemonium. Instead, instructions should be carefully paced and detailed: "Please place your unfinished work on the left side of your desk. (Pause.) Good. Now stand up and push your chairs in—quietly. (Pause.) Very good. Now, first row come and line up at the door."

Such attention to detail is also important when giving the ADHD child directions for academic tasks. The teacher who issues rapid-fire orders is sure to lose the ADHD child in the process. This child needs to have directions stated clearly and simply, one at a time.

INSTEAD OF THIS: "Now it's time to put away your math books and take out your spelling books and a piece of paper. Put your name and the date in the upper right corner of the paper. Then turn to page sixteen in your spelling book and do the first ten words at the bottom of the page."

TRY THIS: "Please close your math books. (Pause to allow ADHD child to follow instruction.) Good. Now put them in your desks. (Pause again.) Now please take out your spelling books. (Pause.) And now take out a piece of paper." And so on.

It's important, too, to be sure that you have the ADHD child's full attention when you give directions. It helps to stand close to the child, perhaps touching his shoulder, to help maintain eye contact and attention.

▪ **Organized materials.** It is vital to ensure that the ADHD child has all of the materials he needs when he leaves the classroom each day. Does this mean that you should check the child's book bag every day before he leaves? Probably not, since this would be a burden for you and an embarrassment to the child. Instead, ask students to raise their hands if they have specific books, then to raise their hands if they have the class handouts, and so on.

Or you might provide the ADHD child with his own "executive secretary"—a well-organized classmate who helps the child gather his materials and ensures that he has everything needed before leaving school.* In every classroom, there is at least one supremely well-organized youngster—usually a girl—who will take such a responsibility seriously and

---

* It's a nice gesture for parents of the ADHD child to recognize the "secretary's" efforts, perhaps with a gift at Christmas or even flowers on Professional Secretaries Day (The Wednesday of the last full week in April).

who can also be counted on to see that the ADHD youngster turns in his completed homework the following day. (In the absence of such an assistant, be sure that you have some other system for collecting homework from the ADHD child, since these children are famous for forgetting to turn in completed work.)

It's also a good idea to schedule housekeeping times when students clean out and reorganize their desks and notebooks. If your ADHD student's "secretary" can help, that's fine. If not, you'll have to provide assistance, because the child certainly can't do it by himself.

Using Feedback to Improve Performance. Like other children, ADHD children benefit most from a combination of negative feedback for errors and positive feedback for appropriate behaviors. To be most effective in promoting learning, a judicious combination of the two should be used.

Unfortunately, like the rest of us, teachers tend to be too stingy with praise and too generous with criticism. Think about it: when was the last time you said, "I really like the way you're paying attention" (instead of "Stop daydreaming and pay attention")? When was the last time you said, "Jeff is working so hard on his project" (instead of "Jeff, get back to work")?

• **Positive Feedback.** Negative feedback is a crazy way to do things in light of the countless studies documenting the power of positive feedback. Study after study paints a consistent picture: when teacher approval (positive feedback) goes up, inappropriate and undesirable behavior goes down.

To help you remember to keep positive feedback at a maximum and negative feedback at a minimum, try the method suggested for parents in Chapter 6. Use an index card divided into columns marked "Praise" and "Criticism" and put a check in the appropriate column every time you praise or criticize a child in your classroom (the ADHD child, or any child, for that matter). Even if you think you're already dispensing lots of positive reinforcement, use this technique to check yourself.

With this information as your baseline, push yourself to give a little more praise and a little less criticism every day. For some this will be fun and easy; others will find it harder. But don't give up because, as your behavior changes, so will the behavior of the children in your class. (In one report, for example, an ADHD child's time on task jumped rapidly from sixty-two percent to ninety-six percent when the teacher switched from criticizing him for off-task behavior to praising him for on-task behavior.)

There are fringe benefits too: not only will you feel better at the end of the day, so will your children. And their behavior will improve, sometimes dramatically. In fact, research shows that you can expect a "spill-over" effect from using lots of positive feedback: even children who aren't the direct recipients of praise show improvement in their behavior when there is lots of praise being dispensed in a classroom.

■ **Negative Feedback.** Negative feedback can't be eliminated entirely, nor should it be, since the best behavior results when ADHD children receive a combination of positive feedback for appropriate behavior and negative feedback for inappropriate behavior. While positive feedback should be delivered loudly and with enthusiasm, negative feedback is best when delivered quietly and unobtrusively. Not only does this spare the ADHD child embarrassment; research shows that negative feedback is most effective when it's delivered privately, quietly, and with a minimum of emotion.[169]

A great way to combine positive and negative feedback is a "response-cost procedure," in which a child earns points for appropriate behavior and loses points for inappropriate behavior. One of the best response-cost systems I've seen for use in the classroom is that devised by Dr. Mark Rapport, a psychologist known for research in ADHD. The do-it-yourself version of Dr. Rapport's system involves two wooden stands with poster-board flip cards consecutively numbered from one to thirty attached. The larger stand, for teacher use, should be visible from anywhere in the classroom if placed on a desk or a chair. The smaller version should fit on the corner of the child's desk.

Using this system, the child can earn a certain amount of free time (up to thirty minutes in Dr. Rapport's program) or points toward another reward by working steadily during independent work time. As the child works, the teacher occasionally checks to see whether he is on task. If not, the teacher will flip a card down and one minute of free time (one point) will be lost.

Teachers find this method simple, practical, and effective. The results, as Dr. Rapport's research shows, are well worth the minimal effort and time spent in constructing the stands, which can be used year after year.

I particularly like the electronic version of Dr. Rapport's method. This cleverly designed system consists of a module on the child's desk that registers points when in operation and a remote-control device that fits in a teacher's pocket. The module registers one point per minute as long as the child is working, but, if the teacher notices that the child is off task, a flick of the button on the remote device causes the module on the child's desk to light up and subtract one point.

This wonderful little gadget is expensive ($330)* but well worth it, since it can be shared among several classrooms, can be used with up to four children at a time, and produces terrific results. Although parents and teachers fear that classmates will ridicule the ADHD child who uses the device, I've found that classmates find the procedure fascinating and soon become an informal cheering squad, especially if the child's success earns a treat for the entire class at the end of the week!

Academics for the ADHD Child

Even ADHD children who do not have learning disabilities have difficulty in the classroom due to their need for physical movement and their problems sustaining attention over time. Dr. Sydney Zentall, a psychologist at Purdue University, has studied the academic performance of ADHD children, and her research over the years has provided a host of valuable guidelines for teachers.[170]

Scheduling. Most ADHD children are more alert and attentive in the morning. Since their attention wanes over the course of the day, the most challenging and demanding academic work should be presented in the morning.

Need for Novelty. Research indicates that ADHD children have what Dr. Zentall calls "an attentional bias toward novelty"; that is, their attention is easily captured by novelty and movement—anything new or different—and drops off dramatically with repetition and familiarity. (This may explain why some ADHD youngsters can hold it together for the first couple of days or weeks in a new school year.)

To meet the ADHD child's need for novelty, tasks should be brief and varied, with immediate feedback for accuracy. Since you, as a teacher,

---

* Attention Training System available from ADD WareHouse (1-800-ADD-WARE).

cannot be everywhere at once in a classroom full of children, you might adopt the strategy of having students check one another's papers at the end of each task.

Format and materials should be varied too. Remember that anything rote is torture for the ADHD child. Unfortunately, some things such as math facts, can be learned only through repetition. For the ADHD child, rote memorization is apt to be less painful and more quickly accomplished when it proceeds at a fast pace and is frequently reinforced. For example, if memorizing math facts is done as a class drill, it should be done in a snappy marching cadence, with plenty of accompanying body movements.

Need for Physical Activity. Even as adults, many ADHD individuals find it painful to sit quietly and passively for long periods of time. These individuals do much better in the classroom when they are provided with frequent breaks for physical activity and when they are allowed to work in an other-than-seated position, if they choose. It goes without saying that the active ADHD youngster should *never* be deprived of recess or sports programs as a punishment for misbehavior, since these children need even more opportunities for movement than other children.

Teachers should also allow fidgety ADHD children to "fiddle" with objects such as beeswax, small sponges, or coated wire while listening to instruction or during "down time" between activities.

The ADHD child also benefits more from any kind of active participation than from passively listening or reading. Thus, ADHD children should be encouraged to underline or highlight as they read, make notes in margins, turn over flash cards, and otherwise interact with the material to be learned.

Helping the ADHD Child with Peer Problems

Whether or not a child is accepted by his classmates can be a make-or-break factor in the child's attitude toward school. And as we've noted repeatedly, ADHD children are often social outcasts in the classroom.

How can you help your ADHD student gain social acceptance? This sounds like a tall order, but, as we've discussed, it's the teacher who sets the tone for the classroom and who can, by example and by direct teaching, encourage all students to behave with courtesy and kindness toward each other.

Indirect Intervention. As a teacher, you can begin by making and enforcing explicit rules for prosocial behavior. Since children are more likely to follow rules they themselves have helped to make, enlist their aid in developing rules for courtesy, cooperation, and prosocial behavior.

Don't make the mistake of thinking that you can do this on a one-shot basis. Instruction needs to be followed up regularly with lots of review, role play, rehearsal, and real-life practice. Catch kids being kind and helpful to each other and call it to the attention of the class. At intervals, ask your students to do a brief self-check of their own prosocial behavior. Encourage positive tattling too: if a child witnesses another student being cooperative and helpful, he should report that to you so that you can praise all parties involved, including the "tattler."

Sounds like a lot of work? No, more like a lot of creativity. And remember: long after the children in your classroom have forgotten how to compute the circumference of a circle, they will remember the safe and caring atmosphere you created for them in your classroom.

Direct Intervention. Encourage other children to include the ADHD child in their activities. With younger children, direct praise is effective: you might say, for example, "Jimmy, I like the way you're sharing the trucks with _____ (ADHD child)." With older children, more subtle expressions of approval are in order. When you see the ADHD child working or playing cooperatively with others, make it a point to comment positively about the activity and the participants. For example, if Ted is engaged in a group project, you can comment on how well everyone is working together and how nicely the project is coming along. Single Ted out for special praise for his contributions.

If the ADHD child has special expertise in an area, call it to the attention of the class. If he has a gift for art, make him the official class artist. If poetry is his strong suit, he can become the class poet laureate. Even if all the child does well is hum rather tunelessly as he works, you can appoint him the class musician and he can be in charge of selecting music to be played during class time (from, of course, a menu of your choosing).

Based on findings from his research, psychologist James Barclay offers these additional suggestions:[171]

- Plan activities in which the ADHD child can participate as an equal or even a superior with other children. For example, have children put on mini-plays, cast the ADHD child in the role of the hero, and commend him for his brilliant performances. (Mini-plays are a delightful teaching device that can be incorporated into the teaching of virtually any subject.)

- Whenever possible, assign choice classroom jobs such as hall patrol, errand runner, or trash monitor* to the ADHD child. Because these coveted positions bestow prestige, the typical practice of giving them to the better students constitutes a flagrant waste of classroom resources. By using these positions to reinforce even small improvements made by the ADHD child, you can reinforce appropriate behavior and, at the same time, confer social status on a child who desperately needs it.

- Break up existing cliques. Don't allow children to form their own groups for projects or other activities. If you do, the popular children will stick together and the less popular ADHD child will be ostracized. Instead, organize groups so that the ADHD child is paired with one or two of the most popular children in the class because popularity tends to "rub off" on others.

Underachievement and Learning Disabilities

As noted in Chapter 2, most youngsters with ADHD have learning difficulties. However, only a relatively small number have the discrepancy between IQ and achievement test scores that by state and federal guidelines entitles them to the full spectrum of special education services within the public schools. Others—many, many others—fall short of this cutoff point and are denied the remedial services that would help them move forward.

* I still haven't figured out what this particular job entails, but I will never forget the day I unknowingly scheduled an appointment for one young patient that prevented him from carrying out his assigned duties in this role. Normally a sunny, sweet youngster who always seemed happy to see me, on this occasion he sulked and pouted through the entire appointment!

Whether or not a child meets an arbitrary cutoff, if he is falling behind in school, an evaluation of his specific difficulties is in order and remedial help is needed. But what constitutes effective "remedial help"? There are so many different types of remedial programs that it's easy to become confused, especially since research on many of these methods is scant or nonexistent.

Indirect Remedial Methods

Training Approaches. In the past, the most widely employed approaches were based on the belief that learning disabilities are caused by underlying perceptual problems or motivational problems. Some of the older indirect approaches, such as the once popular Frostig Program, emphasized training in discriminating visual patterns, forms, and sounds.

Others, like the Doman-Delacato "patterning" method and sensory integrative therapy, use physical exercises and balance training to improve sensory motor functioning. One method, known as optometric vision training, specifically aims to correct the faulty eye movements that supposedly underlie reading problems. Proponents of these approaches argue that training will correct problems in the central nervous system so learning problems will automatically be remedied without other kinds of academic or educational intervention.

Although some of these approaches seem to make sense, none has stood up to the test of rigorous scientific scrutiny. My colleague Sam Goldstein and I reviewed these and other controversial treatments for learning disabilities recently* and concluded that there was little or no solid evidence that they are effective treatments for learning disabilities.

The same is true of remedial approaches that use psychotherapy to treat motivational problems presumed to underlie a child's learning problems. Although psychotherapy may help children and adolescents in other ways, it does not address the learning problems directly so academic gains do not result.

---

* *Attention Deficit Disorder and Learning Disabilities: Realities, Myths and Controversial Treatments.*

Direct Remedial Methods

Direct approaches to remediating learning problems emphasize teaching and practicing the specific skills required for a particular task. For most dyslexic children, for example, effective programs are those that specifically teach letter-sound relationships and sound blending. Two of the better known approaches are the Orton-Gillingham and the DISTAR programs. The Lindamood Auditory Discrimination in Depth program, which teaches phoneme-awareness skills, has been singled out by researchers as particularly promising. The best results are obtained when the instructional package also includes direct instruction in contextual reading.[172]

Programs that improve phonological awareness also can help children who have spelling difficulties, since phonological awareness is an important skill for spelling. Another approach that has been found effective with learning-disabled children is to have the child write incorrectly spelled words correctly several times while simultaneously spelling the word aloud.[173]

Children who have difficulty with the mechanical act of writing—forcing a recalcitrant pencil to produce well-formed, evenly spaced letters—can sometimes benefit from specific programs that teach correct letter formation, size, spacing, and the like. (Some good programs are described later in this chapter.)

Problems with written expression are another matter, since they most commonly involve difficulty organizing one's thoughts. Many youngsters who have such problems find that they are helped by the organizing effects of stimulant medication. Others, however, can benefit from direct instruction in strategies such as semantic maps and "webbing."

It is beyond the scope of this book to describe all the specific approaches that have been found helpful with learning-disabled children, approaches that include strategies training, peer tutoring, and the use of special computer programs. For more information, see the "Resources" section at the end of this chapter.

Special Education Services for ADHD Children

In the not-so-distant past, a child who failed in school was apt to be written off as immature, unmotivated, or simply slow. A popular solution was to have the child repeat the grade. Not surprisingly, this strategy was seldom successful because, without a clear understanding of why the child failed the first time around, the child was usually doomed to fail again.*

Federal Laws and Your Child's Education

With the passage of Public Law 94-142 in 1975, the situation changed considerably for children with handicapping conditions. This law, which was reauthorized in 1990, and again in June 1997, as the Individuals with Disabilities Education Act (IDEA), guarantees a "free and appropriate education" (FAPE) for all handicapped children as well as special services for all handicapped children who need them.

Unfortunately, however, ADHD children were usually denied service under this law unless they had an additional handicapping condition such as a learning disability. Then, in September 1991, thanks to intense lobbying by parent advocacy groups, the U.S. Department of Education issued a memo specifically stating that ADHD children may be eligible for services under the "other health impaired" category of IDEA if the ADHD results in "limited alertness which adversely affects educational performance." Let's take a closer look at this law and what it means for your child's education.

IDEA. Under this law, handicapped children are guaranteed a free and appropriate education; an educational evaluation; an individualized educational plan; placement in the least restrictive environment; parent

---

* Sometimes repeating a grade *can* be beneficial, especially if the child is younger and generally less mature than his classmates. Parents worry that retention will harm a child's self-esteem, but many youngsters jump at the chance for a "catch-up" year.

participation in educational planning; and a right to remedy or due process.

■ **FAPE.** "A free and appropriate education" means that the special services your child needs are provided by the school system at no cost to you. Thus, if the school system cannot provide special services in a public school, they must pay for the child's education in a private school that can provide these services. The key word here, however, is "appropriate": the public school system is not obligated to provide "the best" educational setting, only the most appropriate, and, if they can demonstrate that such a setting is available in a public-school program, they will not pay for placement in a private setting, even though the child might benefit much more over the long term.

■ **Educational Evaluation.** The evaluation process can be initiated either by the parents or by the school but cannot proceed without the parents' written permission. The evaluation must be administered by trained personnel and the evaluation team must be multidisciplinary. However, what constitutes an appropriate evaluation is determined by the school system and, again, that is sometimes a sticking point.

■ **Individualized Educational Plan (IEP).** The IEP is a written plan detailing the program of instruction that will be provided to the child. It is developed at a meeting between parents and school personnel (and, if he wishes to attend, the child himself). All present must jointly agree on what the child's needs are and how services will be provided to meet those needs. The IEP must include the following:

1. A statement of the child's current level of performance in terms of behavior and academic functioning;

2. A statement of annual goals and short-term objectives for each area in which the child has difficulties;

3. A statement of the specific educational and related services to be provided for the child (related services include transportation, speech therapy, occupational therapy, counseling, and the like;

4. The dates services will begin and the expected duration of each service;

5. A description of evaluation procedures to determine whether the objectives are being achieved.

- **Least Restrictive Environment.** Years ago, handicapped children were segregated in special classes or schools that were little more than dumping grounds. Under IDEA, handicapped children must be educated with nonhandicapped children whenever possible. For some children, this means remaining in a regular classroom with resource help and accommodations; others will fare better in special classes or programs.

- **Parent Participation.** Parents must be included as equal partners in developing an educational plan for their children.

In summary, IDEA safeguards the rights of many ADHD children in the school setting. But what if your child does not qualify for services under IDEA? Even children who do not meet the more restrictive criteria of IDEA are often covered under another federal law, known as "Section 504."

Section 504. Section 504 of the Rehabilitation Act of 1973 is a civil rights law that prohibits schools from discriminating against youngsters with disabilities. Under Section 504, a person with disabilities is one "who has a physical or mental impairment which substantially limits a major life activity" (e.g., learning and school performance).

Although eligibility criteria for Section 504 are broader than those for IDEA, not every child with ADHD would be considered eligible for special services as a handicapped person under this law. A bright ADHD youngster, for example, whose attentional difficulties are well controlled on medication and who functions well academically in all areas would certainly not be considered educationally handicapped, nor would he need special services.

However, ADHD children who need accommodations in the regular classroom and/or any other kinds of special services to help them succeed in school are covered under this law and a 504 plan detailing accommodations and special services should be developed. The law does not require a written plan, but I always ask for one because it safeguards against misunderstandings and oversights. It's also helpful to have a written plan when a child changes schools.

Parents As Advocates

To be a successful advocate for your child, you must educate yourself about the federal laws protecting your child's rights. A good starting point is the highly readable and detailed explanation of federal laws and how they apply to your child provided in Chris Dendy's book, *Teenagers with ADD: A Parents' Guide* (see Resources at the end of this chapter).

Other sources of information include articles in newsletters and magazines published by parent support groups. Local chapters often host speakers on topics related to ADHD, and their annual program usually includes at least one talk devoted to educational issues. State, local, and national conferences on ADHD, such as the CH.A.D.D. annual conference, offer informative workshops on how to advocate successfully for your child in the public schools.

Accommodations in the Regular Classroom

About eighty-five to ninety percent of ADHD children can be educated in regular classrooms if they receive accommodations and/or "resource" help.[174] Accommodations most commonly provided for ADHD children include the following:

- Preferential seating, away from doorways and high-traffic areas;
- Home-school assignment sheets initialed by parents and teachers to help with organizational problems;
- Extended time on tests;
- Reduced written work, shortened assignments, and alternatives such as projects in place of written work.

The list of accommodations that can be implemented without undue fuss in the regular classroom is almost endless. For suggestions, see the ADAPT (Attention Deficit Accommodation Plan for Teaching) program and the ADAPT poster developed by Dr. Harvey Parker and *Teenagers with ADD: A Parents' Guide* (see Resources at the end of this chapter).

Accommodations or Excuses? Where do we draw the line between providing accommodations to meet the special needs of an ADHD child and catering to a child who just won't get his act together? There's no pat answer to this question—although you would never know that from the number of people who volunteer advice. Most of this free advice boils down to "Get tough and let him suffer the consequences," a strategy that virtually never works. (Remember, you get what you pay for!)

To put the issue in perspective, think about what your position would be if the child had an orthopedic handicap. Would you be accused of coddling him by allowing him to use a wheelchair or crutches? If he were hearing impaired, would anyone say "He'll be going to high school soon so it's time he started to hear better"?*

Under federal law, ADHD children are entitled to accommodations to help them compensate for handicap-related deficits that interfere with their ability to learn and perform in school. These accommodations aren't meant to give handicapped children an unfair advantage: they're just meant to level the playing field so ADHD children can have a fair shot at success.

Special Class Placement

Some ADHD children—usually those with comorbid psychiatric conditions and/or serious learning disabilities—cannot function successfully in a regular classroom. These children need the highly specialized teaching and small group setting provided only in a self-contained classroom or in a special school.

Parents often fear that if their child is placed in a special education program, he will be locked into special education forever. In this era of tight budgets, nothing could be further from the truth. Every day that a child spends in a special classroom costs the school system money, so you can be sure that the school system will do everything in its power to return a child to the regular classroom as soon as possible.

Before you agree to accept a special education placement for your child, you will have an opportunity to visit the specific classrooms and programs under consideration. Be sure that you can visit while school is in session: looking at an empty classroom won't tell you much about a program. It's particularly important to meet the teacher, since he or she is the critical ingredient in any classroom. Remember that you have the final say concerning your child's placement, so don't give the okay unless

---

* I'm grateful to Patricia Latham at the National Center for Law and Learning Disabilities for this analogy.

you are satisfied that the program is a suitable one for your child. And remember, if you're worried about your child feeling different or ostracized, *your* positive attitude toward the program and intervention and support outside it can make an enormous difference in how a child and his peers perceive this choice.

Home-School Cooperation

Because they see the child under such different circumstances, parents and teachers sometimes have very different perspectives. I am reminded of an instance I cited earlier involving Joey, whose parents reluctantly brought him for an evaluation under pressure from the school. Joey was a charmer, but, charmed as I was, I became increasingly uneasy as he wreaked havoc in my office. Finally, I asked the parents, "Doesn't this behavior bother you at home?" "Oh, no," Joey's mother assured me. "When he gets like this, I just send him out to run around in the yard for a couple of hours. When he comes in, he's a lot calmer."

Obviously, parents and teachers will have very different feelings about Joey's rambunctious behavior. The teacher can't believe that Joey isn't a problem at home, while Joey's mother can't understand why the teacher is making such a fuss. From these very different perspectives, mistrust and animosity grow.

A Working Alliance

How can parents and teachers avoid the trap of mutual blame and mistrust? As a teacher, you can help in the following ways:

■ Remember that the parent has a tremendous emotional investment in the child. Because the parent has so much at stake, emotions may run high. If the parent seems belligerent, try not to take it personally.

■ Remember, too, that parents are in a "one-down" position when they are on your turf. The anxiety this generates may be expressed as defensiveness. Again, don't take it personally.

■ In talking with parents, focus on the child's strengths as much as possible. In describing problems, choose your words carefully and avoid judgmental labels like "irresponsible" and "unmotivated." Stick with factual descriptions of the child's behavior (e.g., "Jake has turned in only four of twelve homework assignments").

Parents, too, must do their share to build a working alliance. As a parent, keep these points in mind:

- Try to understand the teacher's point of view. Behavior that seems inconsequential to you may pose big problems in a class of thirty children.
- When problems crop up, don't automatically side with your child. Because ADHD children have difficulty interpreting the behavior of others toward them, your child's version of a situation may not be an accurate account of what actually happened.
- Be realistic in your expectations. No teacher can be all things to all students. If the teacher can't remember to remind your child to go to the nurse for his medication, for example, work with the teacher, the counselor, and others to develop a workable alternative.

Winning the Homework War

No book on ADHD children would be complete without some reference to this, the bloodiest of all battlegrounds with ADHD children. To parents, the process seems simple enough: bring home your assignments, complete them, and turn in your work the next day. In practice, however, an ADHD child can find a million ways to subvert the process.

He can, for example, forget to write down the assignment or write it incorrectly or forget the necessary books. At home, he procrastinates as long as possible and, once at his desk, he doodles, poodles, and kazoodles around endlessly. When he finally tackles his work, he rushes through, producing a product that is messy, illegible, and full of errors.

Of course, the ADHD child's aversion to homework is understandable. After spending an entire day cooped up in a classroom, he certainly isn't eager for more of the same at home. Nevertheless, homework is a reality of life. What can parents do to help?

■ **Tracking Assignments.** Keeping track of homework assignments is crucial. Sometimes a simple behavior management program is enough: the child earns privileges like television time or computer time by bringing home a list of assignments every day. If he fails to do so, he forfeits his privileges that day.

For the ADHD child who is so disorganized that he can't remember to bring home his assignment list, no matter what the consequences, the teacher or a peer should check the child's assignment notebook at the end of each day. This accommodation should be part of the child's IEP or 504 plan.

For longer-term assignments, provide your child with a month at a glance calendar on which these assignments can be recorded. This gives your child a much better idea of what "due in three weeks" means.

■ **Structuring Time and Space.** Your child should study in an area away from distractions such as siblings, pets, and television. Ideally, he should work at a desk in his bedroom, although with children who require much supervision, this may be a goal rather than a starting point. Whatever the location, there should be no distracting objects nearby—no gerbil cages, no comic books—just the child's work materials.

Set a time when homework is to begin each day. The child should be seated at his workplace, ready to begin, at the established time. Breaks should be scheduled at regular intervals, depending on the individual child. Some children, especially younger ones, need a break every fifteen minutes or so, while older children may need breaks less often.

How much time should a child spend on homework? In the primary grades, fifteen to thirty minutes a day should suffice. By fourth grade, expect about an hour or so. By sixth grade, estimate between one and two hours daily and at least two hours daily by high school.

If your child's homework time often falls far outside these rough limits—your fourth-grader spends three hours daily on homework, for example, or your sixth-grader completes his work in fifteen minutes—something's wrong. The dawdler is probably wasting time, while the speed demon is almost certainly producing sloppy, half-finished work.

Knowing that he must remain at his desk for a fixed period of time regardless of whether he finishes early helps slow down the speedster. The slowpoke, on the other hand, can benefit from methods that boost time-on-task.

■ **Maximizing Time-on-Task.** An excellent way to help ADHD children stay on task is to use an "attention tape," an audiotape that has soft tones at intervals.* He starts the tape when he begins his homework. Each time he hears a tone, he asks himself, "Was I on task?" If the answer is yes, he checks the "Yes" column on a sheet of paper. Otherwise, he makes a check in the "No" column.

For the most part, children with whom I've used this method have found it helpful and fun. Parents agree that it helps children stay on task, so work is completed faster and more accurately.

Winning the Battle, Losing the War

For many ADHD children, simple interventions such as those described above will result in marked reductions in homework problems. For some, however, nothing seems to work, and by the teen years, screaming battles over homework and grades tear at the very fabric of family life.

If this has happened in your family, it's time to call a halt and take a long, hard look at the problem. Perhaps, in addition to his attentional and organizational problems, your child has learning disabilities that have gone undetected. Even if an educational evaluation in the past did not seem to indicate such problems, don't be too quick to rule them out: in my practice, I have seen many young people whose early test results should have been a red flag, alerting parents and teachers to difficulties. Somehow these red flags went unrecognized and the child's performance went from poor to abysmal over the years. For some of these youngsters, I've found that appropriate accommodations and remedial measures can make a big difference in school performance.

Or perhaps your child would fare better in a different school. So-called "alternative" schools have their drawbacks, but for some young people, they offer a lifeline. One young patient of mine was able to complete an

---

* "Listen, Look, and Think" tape available from ADD WareHouse (1-800-ADD-WARE).

entire year in a single semester at such a school. Another patient, highly gifted but quite learning disabled, described his experience in an alternative school quite simply: "They saved my life."

As a first step in your deliberations, make an appointment to consult with an educational placement specialist or a clinical psychologist who is knowledgeable about both ADHD and learning problems. These professionals can help you obtain appropriate evaluations and can guide you and your child toward greater educational success.

Resources for Parents and Teachers

Most of the books listed below are available in local bookstores or through the ADD WareHouse (1-800-ADD-WARE). For others, call the telephone number provided.

Bradley-Johnson, S., and J. Lesiak. *Problems in Written Expression*. New York: Guilford Press, 1989.

Canter, L., and L. Hausner. *Homework Without Tears*. New York: Harper, 1987.

Dendy, C. *Teenagers with ADD: A Parents' Guide*. Bethesda, Md.: Woodbine House, 1995. (1-800-843-7323).

DuPaul, G. J., and G. Stoner. *ADHD in the Schools: Assessment and Intervention Strategies*. New York: Guilford Press, 1994.

Fowler, M. *CH.A.D.D. Educators Manual*. Fairfax, Va.: Caset Associates, 2nd ed., 1995. (1-800-545-5583).

Goldstein, S. *Understanding and Managing Children's Classroom Behavior*. New York: John Wiley, 1995.

NICHD. *Learning Disabilities/Reading Disabilities Information Packet: Research Discoveries—Clinical Applications*. No charge; available from the National Institute of Child Health and Human Development/NIH; Learning Disabilities, Cognitive and Social Development Branch, 6100 Executive Boulevard, Room 4B05G, Rockville, MD 20852.

Parker, H. C. *The ADD Hyperactivity Handbook for Schools*. Plantation, Fla.: Impact Publications, 1991 (ADD WareHouse: 1-800-233-9273).

Radencich, M., and J. S. Schumm. *How to Help Your Child with Home-*

work. Minneapolis, Minn.: Free Spirit Publishing (1–612–338–2068), 1988.

Reif, S. *How to Reach and Teach ADD/ADHD Children*. West Nyack, N.Y.: The Center for Applied Research in Education, 1993.

Vail, P. *Smart Kids with School Problems*. New York: Plume/Penguin, 1987.

CHAPTER 10

THE DECADE AHEAD

What Can We Expect?

In the past decade, there have been so many advances in our knowledge about ADHD that we have every right to be optimistic about how children and adults with ADHD will fare in the years ahead. There are, however, still some obstacles to overcome and a lot of painstaking work to be done along the way.

I don't have access to the proverbial crystal ball. Nevertheless, based on what I know about ADHD, I will hazard some guesses about what the future holds for individuals with ADHD.

Diagnosis

The Good News

We can expect that advances in technology will result in more precise information about the specific brain areas and neurotransmitters involved in ADHD. Using newer brain imaging techniques, computerized EEGs, and methods for assessing neurotransmitter activity in the living brain, neuroscientists will be able to define subtypes of ADHD with much greater precision than is now the case. These advances should also allow us to identify comorbid conditions as well.

As Dr. Russell Barkley notes, there is also reason to believe that advances on the genetic front will add to our knowledge base. If we can identify the gene or genes associated with ADHD, we would have a genetic "marker" that would aid enormously in diagnosis.

Such a genetic marker would also help us identify at-risk children at a very early age so that we could put preventive programs in place. As in virtually every other condition you can think of, it's quite likely that the adage "An ounce of prevention is worth a pound of cure" will hold true in ADHD also. Dr. Barkley, who is conducting an early-intervention program with kindergarten children who are at high risk for ADHD, is optimistic that programs such as his will reduce the educational and social risks these children face and improve the outcome for all youngsters with ADHD.[175]

The Work Ahead

We must remember, however, that the research needed to achieve these goals is expensive and that tax dollars needed to fund this research are scarce. At the National Institute of Mental Health, scientists and administrators who conduct and fund this all-important research worry constantly about budget cuts that will force them to curtail research efforts. Thus, there was great relief when, after the budget crisis of 1996, funding for each division at NIMH was actually increased by more than five percent.[176] However, while funding for ADHD research is expected to do well in the immediate future, there is always the risk that it could be slashed in the next round of budget cutbacks and cost-cutting. Consumer groups such as CH.A.D.D., ADDA, and AMI-CAN★ lobby actively to increase funding for research in ADHD and other psychiatric disorders— just one more reason for you as a parent to become active in these groups.

★ Alliance for the Mentally Ill—Children and Adolescents Network. See Appendix B.

Treatment

The Good News

When we achieve greater diagnostic precision, we can look forward to treatment plans tailored to meet the needs of each individual. For example, as Dr. Pat Quinn has observed, we might find that ADHD youngsters with low levels of metabolic activity in the frontal areas of the brain respond best to stimulant medication, while ADHD individuals with other patterns of brain activity respond better to alternative medications.[177]

Greater diagnostic precision will also help us determine just what kinds of treatments and interventions will be most beneficial to each ADHD child, adolescent, and adult. Findings from such ambitious research programs as the six-site Multi-Modal Treatment of Attention-Deficit/Hyperactivity Disorder Study sponsored by NIMH will enable us to determine which children need adjunctive treatments in addition to medication. Findings from these studies will also help us identify youngsters who need only a single intervention, such as medication or parent training.

I think that we can also expect advances in the area of psychopharmacology. I look forward to new medicines which are targeted more precisely at specific symptom patterns and are also less likely to produce unwanted side effects. With so many ADHD individuals now being treated with medication, there is an expanded market for better medicines. As an example, Richwood Pharmaceutical Company recently introduced the stimulant Adderal for treatment of ADHD. It's likely that potential profits from new and improved medications will encourage other drug companies to devote energy and effort toward developing other new medicines for ADHD.

The Work Ahead

On the other hand, the profit motive in the form of so-called "managed health care" will probably continue to make it difficult or impossible for many children and adults with ADHD to receive the thorough diagnostic workup and systematic follow-up services they need. Speaking as president of the American Psychiatric Association, Dr. Harold Eist recently described the managed-care industry as "rapacious, dishonest, destructive, [and] greed-driven." Managed care, he added, is "in the process of decimating all health care in America, particularly . . . the care of the mentally ill."[178]

While many professionals believe that managed care is inevitable, there are also many who disagree and who, like Dr. Eist, have taken a stand against the invasion of managed care. Lawsuits have been filed against managed care companies in several states. Professionals and consumers have joined ranks in an organization called the National Coalition of Mental Health Professionals and Consumers.* As a consumer of mental health services, you might want to join this organization to help you understand your rights and to learn how you can fight the limits your managed-care plan places on your ability to obtain the services your child needs.

I believe that managed care companies have specifically targeted mental health benefits for "management" not because these benefits are so costly (since the data clearly debunk this notion), but because people with psychiatric problems are often reluctant to fight back, fearing the stigma that many associate with these conditions. However, the media coverage that has resulted in increased public awareness has had the additional benefit of removing much of the stigma associated with ADHD, at least. Therefore, parents of ADHD children as well as adults with the disorder now feel more comfortable complaining to an employer about the lack of mental health services in insurance plans offered by that employer.

And that is what you need to do—complain, speak up, speak out to those who can do something about the problem. In the long run, I do not think that managed care will prevail, but it will take our united efforts to fight it.

* P. O. Box 438, Commack, NY 11725–0438 (Phone/fax 1-516-424-5232).

On the School Front

The Good News

From the foregoing, it is clear that I am optimistic about our ability to help individuals with ADHD succeed at home, in school, and in the workplace. Progress has certainly been made in educating teachers about how to identify and work with ADHD children. In fact, I've been surprised and gratified by the level of sophistication and knowledge I've observed in elementary school teachers in recent years. Elementary-school guidance counselors have also become much more knowledgeable about ADHD and many have taken the initiative to provide special services such as "friendship groups" for ADHD youngsters who are struggling with academic and social problems.

I'm encouraged, too, by the recent advances in our knowledge about learning disabilities and the new techniques and technologies that promise to be of help to learning-disabled children with and without ADHD. We've only begun to explore the wonderful possibilities that computers can offer in the way of helping learning-disabled children, for example, and it's likely that what is now a trickle in terms of computerized remedial programs will soon become a flood.

The Work Ahead

Unfortunately, however, I've found that while elementary-school teachers have profited from training to identify and work with ADHD children, many middle-school and high-school teachers remain woefully undereducated concerning ADHD. Clearly, there is a pressing need to provide in-service training to teachers in these settings. Again, however, budget cutbacks make it unlikely that appropriate training will be offered to these professionals. It is my hope that CH.A.D.D. and other parent support groups will rally to the cause and will work with local school systems to find ways to meet this need.

For the immediate future, things do not bode well for ADHD youngsters in the public schools, even at the elementary level. This is an age of budget cutbacks in the public school system, and for the next few years, at least, I think that will continue to encounter resistance on the part of public schools toward providing comprehensive assessments and special education services. Certainly, there will be reluctance on the part of school systems across the country to fund placements for ADHD children in expensive schools that specialize in working with children with ADHD and/or learning disabilities.

The Last Word

After twenty-eight years of working with ADHD children and their families, I am deeply gratified to see the progress that has been made over the last quarter of a century. As a clinician and an advocate for youngsters with ADHD, I can't wait to see what new knowledge unfolds in the coming years—and I'm excited about summarizing this knowledge in another book a decade from now!

Appendix A

Developmental and Social History

Child's name _____ Date of birth _____

School _____ Grade _____

School address _____

Teacher's name _____ School phone# _____

Father's name _____ Mother's name _____

Education _____ Education _____

Occupation _____ Occupation _____

Are parents still married? Yes _____ No _____

Other children in family Age Personal/social/academic adjustment

_____ _____ _____

_____ _____ _____

_____ _____ _____

Prenatal:

Problems during pregnancy, labor, delivery _____

_____

Note any problems with: feeding _____ vomiting _____ crying _____

colic _____ diarrhea _____ Other _____

_____

Early Development:

Gross motor development (sitting, standing, walking) was:

early _____ normal range _____ late _____

Fine motor skills developed:

early _____ normal range _____ late _____

Speech/language development was:

early _____ normal range _____ late _____

Bowel/bladder training was:

early _____ normal range _____ late _____

If there were problems in any of these areas, please describe: _____

_____

_____

Medical History:

Does child have a history of chronic ear/respiratory infections, allergies, other illnesses?   (Please explain) _____

_____

_____

_____

School History:

Please describe child's behavioral and academic performance ·in:

PRESCHOOL _____

_____

_____

ELEMENTARY SCHOOL _____

_____

_____

MIDDLE SCHOOL _____

_____

_____

HIGH SCHOOL _____

_____

_____

Personal Relationships:

How does child get along with each parent? _____

_____

_____

How does child get along with siblings? _____

_____

_____

How does child get along with friends? _____

_____

_____

Habits:

If child has had problems in any of the following areas, please describe below:

   —school failure

   —temper tantrums, irritable moods

   —poor frustration tolerance

   —restlessness, hyperactivity

   —problems with attention, concentration

   —physical ailments (stomachaches, headaches, etc.)

   —fear of leaving parents

   —other significant fears

   —insomnia, interrupted sleep, nightmares

   —stealing, lying

   —cruelty to peers, animals

   —destruction of property

   —physical aggression, fighting

   —sadness, low moods

   —fatigue, low energy

   —drug, alcohol use

   —chronic boredom, lack of enthusiasm/fun

Problem descriptions: _____

_____

_____

_____

_____

Family History:

Among the child's blood relatives, including grandparents, aunts, and uncles, is there anyone who has had learning problems, hyperactivity, depression, anxiety disorders, drug abuse, or alcoholism?

_____

_____

_____

For what problems are you seeking help right now?

_____

_____

If your child has had treatment for these problems, please describe. _____

_____

_____

Other Concerns:

Please describe any other concerns not directly addressed in this questionnaire. _____

_____

_____

Appendix B

ADHD Support Services

For additional information on chapters in your area and other sources of support, contact the following national organizations serving the ADHD community:

CH.A.D.D. (Children and Adults with Attention Deficit Disorders)
499 Northwest 70th Avenue
Suite 109
Plantation, FL 33317
1-305-587-3700 or 1-800-233-4050

ADDA (National Attention Deficit Disorder Association)
P. O. Box 972
Mentor, OH 44061
1-216-350-9595 or 1-800-487-2282

AADF (Adult Attention Deficit Foundation)
132 North Woodward Avenue
Birmingham, MI 48009
1-810-540-6335

AMI-CAN (Alliance for the Mentally Ill—Children and Adolescents
Network)
200 N. Glebe Road, Suite 1015
Arlington, VA 22203
1-703-524-7600

NOTES

1. American Psychiatric Association. *Diagnostic and Statistical Manual of Mental Disorders*. Washington, D.C.: American Psychiatric Association, 1994.

2. Barkley, R. A. *Hyperactive Children: A Handbook for Diagnosis and Treatment*. New York: Guilford Press, 1981, passim.

3. Barkley, R. A. "A new theory of ADHD." *ADHD Report*. 1994, 1 (5), 1–4.

4. Biederman, J., Faraone, S., Milberger, S., Curtis, S., Chen, L., Marrs, A., Ouellette, C., Moore, P., and T. Spencer. "Predictors of persistence and remission of ADHD into adolescence: Results from a four-year prospective follow-up study." *American Journal of Child and Adolescent Psychiatry*. 1996, 35, 343–351.

5. Barkley, R. A. "ADD research: A look at today and tomorrow." Interview. *Attention*. 3, 1996, 9–11.

6. Nada-Raja, S., Langley, J. D., McGee, R., Williams, S. M., Begg, D. J., and A. J. Reeder. "Inattentive and hyperactive behaviors and driving offenses in adolescence." *Journal of the American Academy of Child and Adolescent Psychiatry*. 1997, 36, 515–522.

7. Barkley, R. A., Fischer, M., Edelbrock, C. S., and L. Smallish. "The Adolescent Outcome of Hyperactive Children Diagnosed by Research Criteria:

I. An 8-Year Prospective Follow-up Study." *Journal of the American Academy of Child and Adolescent Psychiatry.* 1990, 29, 546–557.

8. Mantzicopoulos, P. Y., and D. Morrison. "A Comparison of Boys and Girls with Attention Problems: Kindergarten through Second Grade." *American Journal of Orthopsychiatry.* 1994, 64, 522–533.

9. Schaughency, E., McGee, R., Raja, S. N., Feehan, M., and P. A. Silva. "Self-reported inattention, impulsivity, and hyperactivity at ages 15 and 18 years in the general population." *Journal of the American Academy of Child and Adolescent Psychiatry.* 1994, 33, 173–184.

10. Gallucci, F., Bird, H., Berardi, C., Gallai, V., Pfanner, P., and A. Weinberg. "Symptoms of Attention-Deficit Hyperactivity Disorder in an Italian school sample: Findings of a pilot study." *Journal of the American Academy of Child and Adolescent Psychiatry.* 1993, 32, 1051–1058.

11. Williams, L., Lerner, M., Wigal, T., and J. Swanson. "Minority Assessment of ADD: Issues in the Development of New Assessment Techniques." *Attention.* 2, 1, 9–15.

12. Murphy, K. R. "Coping Strategies for ADHD Adults." *CH.A.D.D.ER.* 1992, 6, 2, 10.

13. Barkley, R. A., DuPaul, G. J., and M. B. McMurray. "Comprehensive evaluation of attention deficit disorder with and without hyperactivity as defined by research criteria." *Journal of Consulting and Clinical Psychology.* 1990, 58, 775–789.

14. Lahey, B. B., and C. L. Carlson. "Validity of the diagnostic category of attention deficit disorder without hyperactivity." *Journal of Learning Disabilities.* 1991, 24, 110–120.

15. Paternite, C. E., Loney, J., and M. A. Roberts. "A preliminary validation of subtypes of DSM-IV attention-deficit/hyperactivity disorder." *Journal of Attention Disorders.* 1996, 1, 70–86.

16. Seidman, L. J., Biederman, J., Faraone, S. V., Milberger, S., Norman, D., Seiverd, K., Benedict, K., Guite, J., Mick, E., and K. Kiely. "Effects of Family History and Comorbidity on the Neuropsychological Performance of Children with ADHD: Preliminary Findings." *Journal of the American Academy of Child and Adolescent Psychiatry.* 1995, 34, 1015–1024.

17. Cantwell, D. P. "Attention deficit disorder: A review of the past 10 years." *Journal of the American Academy of Child and Adolescent Psychiatry.* 1996, 35, 978–987.

18. Maziade, M. "Should Adverse Temperament Matter to the Clinician? An Empirically Based Answer." In Kohnstamm, G. A., Bates, J. E., and M. K. Rothbart, eds. *Temperament in Childhood.* New York: John Wiley, 1989, passim.

19. Wenning, K., Nathan, P., and S. King. "Mood disorders in children with

Oppositional Defiant Disorder: A pilot study." *American Journal of Orthopsychiatry.* 1993, 63, 295–299.

20. McBurnett, K. "ADD and Delinquency: Myths, Pathways, and Advice." *Attention.* 1996, 2, 20–26.

21. Kovacs, M., and Gatsonis, C. "Stability and change in childhood-onset depressive disorders: Longitudinal course as a diagnostic validator." In Robins, L. N., and J. E. Barrett, eds. *The Validity of Psychiatric Diagnosis.* New York: Raven Press, 1989, pp. 57–76.

22. Winokur, G., Coryell, W., Endicott, J., and H. Akiskal. "Further distinctions between manic-depressive illness (bipolar disorder) and primary depressive disorder (unipolar depression)." *American Journal of Psychiatry.* 1993, 150, 1176–1181.

23. Regier, D. A., Boyd, J. H., Burke, J. D., Rae, D. S., Myers, J. K., Kramer, M., Robins, L. M., Georgia, L. K., Karno, M., and B. Z. Locke. "One-month prevalence of mental disorders in the United States: Based on five epidemiologic-catchment area sites." *Archives of General Psychiatry.* 1988, 45, 977–986.

24. McCauley, E., Myers, K., Mitchell, J., Calderon, R., Schloredt, K., and R. Treder. "Depression in young people: Initial presentation and clinical course." *Journal of the American Academy of Child and Adolescent Psychiatry.* 1993, 32, 714–722.

25. Perrin, S., and C. G. Last. "Relationship between ADHD and anxiety in boys: Results from a family study." *Journal of the American Academy of Child and Adolescent Psychiatry.* 1996, 35, 988–996.

26. Nolan, E. E., Sverd, J., Gadow, K. D., Sprafkin, J., and S. N. Ezor. "Associated psychopathology in children with both ADHD and chronic tic disorder." *Journal of the American Academy of Child and Adolescent Psychiatry.* 1996, 35, 1622–1630.

27. Vail, P. *Smart Kids with School Problems.* New York: Penguin/Plume, 1987, passim.

28. Faraone, S. V., Biederman, J., Lehman, B., Spencer, T., Norman, D., Seidman, L., Kraus, P., Perrin, J., Chen, W., and M. Tsuang. "Intellectual performance and school failure in children with attention-deficit/hyperactivity disorder and their siblings." *Journal of Abnormal Psychology.* 1993, 102, 616–623.

29. Barkley, R. A. *Attention-Deficit/Hyperactivity Disorder: A Handbook for Diagnosis and Treatment.* New York: Guilford Press, 1990, p. 88.

30. Cantwell, D. P., and L. Baker. "Attention deficit disorder with and without hyperactivity: A review and comparison of matched groups." *Journal of the American Academy of Child and Adolescent Psychiatry.* 1992, 31, 432–438.

31. Riccio, C. A., Hynd, G. W., Cohen, M. J., Hall, J., and L. Molt. "Comorbidity of Central Auditory Processing Disorder and Attention-Deficit

Hyperactivity Disorder." *Journal of the American Academy of Child and Adolescent Psychiatry.* 1994, 33, 849–857.

32. Tannock, R., Purvis, K. L., and R. J. Schachar. "Narrative abilities in children with Attention-Deficit/Hyperactivity Disorder and normal peers." *Journal of Abnormal Child Psychology.* 1993, 21, 103–117.

33. Beitchman, J. H., Wilson, B., Brownlie, E. B., Walters, H., and W. Lancee. "Long-term Consistency in Speech/Language profiles: I. Developmental and Academic Outcomes." *Journal of the American Academy of Child and Adolescent Psychiatry.* 1996, 804–814.

34. Naylor, M. W., Staskowski, M., Kenney, M. C., and C. A. King. "Language Disorders and Learning Disabilities in School-Refusing Adolescents." *Journal of the American Academy of Child and Adolescent Psychiatry.* 1994, 1331–1337.

35. Adesman, A.R.A., Altshuler, L. A., Lipkin, P. H., and G. A. Walco. "Otitis media in children with learning disabilities and in children with attention deficit disorder with hyperactivity." *Pediatrics.* 1990, 85, 442–446.

36. Warren, R. P., Odell, J. D., Warren, W., Burger, R. A., Maciulis, A., and A. R. Torres. "Is decreased blood plasma concentration of the complement C4B protein associated with Attention-Deficit Hyperactivity Disorder?" *Journal of the American Academy of Child and Adolescent Psychiatry.* 1995, 34, 1009–1014.

37. Daly, J. M., Biederman, J., Bostic, J. Q., Maraganore, A. M., Lelon, E., Jellinek, M. P., and A. Lapey. "The Relationship Between Childhood Asthma and Attention-Deficit/Hyperactivity Disorder: A Review of the Literature." *Journal of Attention Disorders.* 1996, 1, 31–40.

38. Deutsch, C. K., Matthysse, S., Swanson, J. M., and L. G. Frakas. "Genetic latent structure analysis of dysmorphology in Attention Deficit Disorder." *Journal of the American Academy of Child and Adolescent Psychiatry.* 1990, 29, 189–194.

39. La Greca, A. M., and M. D. Fetter. "Peer relations." In A. R. Eisen, C. A. Kearney, and C. E. Schaefer, eds. *Clinical Handbook of Anxiety Disorders in Children and Adolescents.* Northvale, N.J.: Jason Aronson, Inc., 1995, 83.

40. Barkley, R. A. "Can neuropsychological tests help diagnose ADD/ADHD?" *ADHD Report.* 1994, 2, 1–3.

41. Seidman, L. J., Biederman, J., Faraone, S. V., Milberger, S., Norman, D., Seiverd, K., Benedict, K., Guite, J., Mick, E., and K. Kiely. "Effects of family history and comorbidity on the neuropsychological performance of children with ADHD: Preliminary findings." *Journal of the American Academy of Child and Adolescent Psychiatry.* 1995, 34, 1015–1024.

42. American Academy of Neurology. "Role of neurodiagnostic testing questioned in ADHD." *American Academy of Neurology AANews.* 1993, 6, 6.

43. Brown, T. E. *Brown Attention-Deficit Disorder Scales*. San Antonio: The Psychological Corp., 1996, passim.

44. Murphy, K., and R. A. Barkley. "Updated Adult Norms for the ADHD Behavior Checklist for Adults." *The ADHD Report*. 1996, 4, 12.

45. Hartmann, T., *Attention Deficit Disorder: A Different Perception*. Grass Valley, Cal.: Underwood Books, 1993, passim.

46. Barkley, R. A., and C. E. Cunningham. "The parent-child interactions of hyperactive children and their modification by stimulant drugs." In Knights, R. and D. Bakker, eds. *Treatment of Hyperactive and Learning Disabled Children*. Baltimore: University Park Press, 1980, pp. 219–236.

47. Chess, S., and A. Thomas. *Temperament in Clinical Practice*. New York: Guilford Press, 1986, passim.

48. Chess, S. and A. Thomas. *Temperament in Clinical Practice*. New York: Guilford Press, 1986, p. 30.

49. Maziade Psychiatric Development, 1988.

50. Hartsough, C. S., and N. M. Lambert. "Medical factors in hyperactive and normal children: Prenatal, developmental, and health history findings." *American Journal of Orthopsychiatry*. 1985, 55, 190–210.

51. Sprich-Buckminster, S., Biederman, J., Milberger, S., Faraone, S. V., and B. K. Lehman. "Are perinatal complications relevant to the manifestation of ADD? Issues of comorbidity and familiality." *Journal of the American Academy of Child and Adolescent Psychiatry*. 1993, 32, 1032–1037.

52. Schothorst, P. F., and H. van Engeland. "Long-term behavioral sequelae of prematurity." *Journal of the American Academy of Child and Adolescent Psychiatry*. 1996, 35, 175–183.

53. American Academy of Pediatrics, Committee on Substance Abuse. "Fetal alcohol syndrome and fetal alcohol effects." *Pediatrics*. 1993, 91, 1004–1006.

54. Milberger, S., Biederman, J., Faraone, S. V., Chen, L., and J. Jones. "Is maternal smoking during pregnancy a risk factor for Attention-Deficit/Hyperactivity Disorder in children?" *American Journal of Psychiatry*. 1996, 153, 1138–1142.

55. Conners, C. K., Levin, E. D., Sparrows, E., Hinton, S. C., Erhardt, D., Meck, W. H., Rose, J. E., and J. March. "Nicotine and attention in adult Attention-Deficit/Hyperactivity Disorder (ADHD)." *Psychopharmacology Bulletin*. 1996, 32, 67–83.

56. Scherling, D. "Prenatal cocaine exposure and childhood psychopathology: A developmental analysis." *American Journal of Orthopsychiatry*. 1994, 64, 9–19.

57. Needelman, H. L., Reiss, J. A., Tobin, M. J., Biesecker, G. E., and J. B.

Greenhouse. "Bone lead levels and delinquent behavior." *Journal of the American Medical Association.* 1996, 275, 363–369.

58. Burd, L., Kerbeshian, J., and W. Fisher. "Does the use of phenobarbital as an anticonvulsant permanently exacerbate hyperactivity?" *Canadian Journal of Psychiatry.* 1987, 32, 10–13.

59. Bennett, F. C., and R. Sherman. "Management of childhood 'hyperactivity' by primary care physicians." *Journal of Developmental and Behavioral Pediatrics.* 1983, 4, 88–93.

60. Conners, C. K. *Feeding the Brain: How Foods Affect Children.* New York: Plenum Press, 1989, p. 99.

61. Biederman, J., Faraone, S. V., Mick, E., Spencer, T., Wilens, T., Kiely, K., Guite, J., Ablon, J. S., Reed, E., and R. Warburton. "High risk for Attention-Deficit/Hyperactivity Disorder among children of parents with childhood onset of the disorder: A pilot study." *American Journal of Psychiatry.* 1995, 152, 431–435.

62. Faraone, S. V., and J. Biederman. "Is Attention-Deficit/Hyperactivity Disorder Familial?" *Harvard Review of Psychiatry.* 1994, 39, 271–287.

63. Gillis, J. J., Gilger, J. W., Pennington, B. F., and J. C. DeFries. "Attention Deficit Disorder in Reading Disabled Twins: Evidence for a Genetic Etiology." *Journal of Abnormal Child Psychology.* 1992, 20, 303–315.

64. Goodman, R., and J. Stevenson. "A Twin Study of Hyperactivity: II. The Aetiological Role of Genes, Family Relationships, and Perinatal Adversity." *Journal of Child Psychology and Psychiatry.* 1989, 30, 691–709.

65. Cantwell, D. P. *The Hyperactive Child: Diagnosis, Management, Current Research.* New York: Spectrum, 1975.

66. Alberts-Corush, J., Firestone, P., and J. T. Goodman. "Attention and impulsivity characteristics of the biological and adoptive parents of hyperactive and normal control children." *American Journal of Orthopsychiatry.* 1986, 56, 413–423.

67. McInnis, M. G., McMahon, F. J., Chase, G. A., Simpson, S. G., Ross, C. A., and J. R. DePaulo. "Anticipation in bipolar affective disorder." *American Journal of Human Genetics.* 1993, 53, 385–390.

68. Gorwood, P., Leboyer, M., Falissard, B., Jay, M., Rouillon, F., and J. Feingold. "Anticipation in schizophrenia: New light on a controversial problem." *American Journal of Psychiatry.* 1996, 153, 1173–1177.

69. Warren, R. P., Odell, J. D., Warren, W. L., Burger, R. A., Maciulis, A., and A. R. Torres. "Is decreased blood plasma concentration of the complement C4B protein associated with Attention-Deficit/Hyperactivity Disorder?" *Journal of the American Academy of Child and Adolescent Psychiatry.* 1995, 343, 1009–1014.

70. Odell, J. D., Warren, R. P., Warren, W. L., Burger, R. A., and A.

Maciulis. "Association of genes within the major histocompatibility complex with Attention-Deficit/Hyperactivity Disorder." *Neuropsychobiology*. in press.

71. Castellanos, F. X., Giedd, H. N., Marsh, W. L., Hamburger, S. D., Vaituzis, A. C., Dickstein, D. P., Sarfatti, S. E., Vauss, Y. C., Snell, J. W., Rajapakse, J. C., and J. L. Rapoport. "Quantitative brain magnetic resonance imaging in Attention-Deficit/Hyperactivity Disorder." *Archives of General Psychiatry*. 1996, 53, 607–616.

72. Castellanos, F. X. "Toward a pathophysiology of Attention-Deficit/Hyperactivity Disorder." *Clinical Pediatrics*. in press.

73. Kuperman, S., Johnson, B., Arndt, S., Lindgren, S., and M. Wolraich. "Quantitative EEG Differences in a Nonclinical Sample of Children with ADHD and Undifferentiated ADD." *Journal of the American Academy of Child and Adolescent Psychiatry*. 1996, 35, 1009–1017.

74. Lou, H. C., Hendricksen, L., and P. Bruhn. "Focal cerebral hypoperfusion in children with dysphasia and/or attention deficit disorder." *Archives of Neurology*. 1984, 41, 825–829.

75. Zametkin, A. J., Nordahl, T. E., Gross, M., King, A. C., Semple, W. E., Rumsey, J., Hamburger, S., and R. M. Cohen. "Cerebral glucose metabolism in adults with hyperactivity of childhood onset." *New England Journal of Medicine*. 1990, 323, 1361–1366.

76. Castellanos, F. X., Elia, J., Kruesi, M.J.P., Marsh, W. L., Gulotta, C. S., Potter, W. Z., Ritchie, G. F., Hamburger, S. D., and J. L. Rapoport. "Cerebrospinal fluid homovanillic acid predicts behavioral response to stimulants in 45 boys with Attention-Deficit/Hyperactivity Disorder." *Neuropsychopharmacology*. 1996, 14, 125–137.

77. Benjamin, J., Li, L., Patterson, C., Greenberg, B. D., Murphy, D. L., and D. H. Hamer. "Population and familial association between the D4 dopamine receptor gene and measures of novelty seeking." *Nature Genetics*. 1996, 12, 81–84.

78. Cook, E. H., Stein, M. A., Krasowski, M. D., Cox, N. J., Olkon, D. M., Kieffer, J. E., and B. L. Leventhal. "Association of Attention-Deficit Disorder and the dopamine transporter gene." *American Journal of Human Genetics*. 1995, 56, 993–998.

79. Mannuzza, S., Klein, R. G., Bessler, A., Malloy, P., and M. LaPadula. "Adult outcome of hyperactive boys. Educational achievement, occupational rank, and psychiatric status." *Archives of General Psychiatry*. 1993, 50, 565–576.

80. Barkley, R. A. *Taking Charge of ADHD*. New York: Guilford Press, 1995, p. 65.

81. Barkley, R. A. "An interview with John Werry." *Attention*. 1995, 2, 1, 30.

82. Jensen, P. S. "Evolution and revolution in child psychopathology: ADHD and child psychopathology as disorders of adaptation." *Journal of the American Academy of Child and Adolescent Psychiatry*. in press.

83. Safer, D. J. "Medication usage trends for ADD." *Attention*. 1995, 2, 11–15.

84. Hunt, R. Study cited in *Child and Adolescent Psychopharmacology News*. 1996, 1, 7.

85. Elia, J., Borcherding, B. G., Rapoport, J. L., and C. S. Keysor. "Methylphenidate and dextroamphetamine treatments of hyperactivity: Are there true nonresponders?" *Psychiatry Research*. 1991, 36, 141–155.

86. Keith, R. W., and P. Engineer. "Effects of methylphenidate on the auditory processing abilities of children with attention-deficit-hyperactivity disorder." *Journal of Learning Disabilities*. 1991, 24, 630–636, 640.

87. Tannock, R., Fine, J., Heintz, T., and R. J. Schachar. "A linguistic approach detects stimulant effects in two children with Attention-Deficit/Hyperactivity Disorder." *Journal of Child and Adolescent Psychopharmacology*. 1995, 5, 177–189.

88. O'Toole, K., Abramowitz, A., Morris, R., and M. Dulcan. "Effects of methylphenidate on attention and nonverbal learning in children with Attention-Deficit/Hyperactivity Disorder." *Journal of the American Academy of Child and Adolescent Psychiatry*. 1997, 36, 531–538.

89. Rapport, M. D., Denney, C., DuPaul, G. J., and M. J. Gardner. "Attention Deficit Disorder and Methylphenidate: Normalization Rates, Clinical Effectiveness, and Response Prediction in 76 Children." *Journal of the American Academy of Child and Adolescent Psychiatry*. 1994, 33, 882–93.

90. Pelham, W. E., Bender, M. A., Caddell, J., Booth, S., and S. H. Moorer. "Methylphenidate and children with Attention Deficit Disorder: Dose effects on classroom academic and social behavior." *Archives of General Psychiatry*. 1985, 42, 948–52.

91. Stephens, R. S., Pelham, W. E., and R. Skinner. "State-dependent and main effects of methylphenidate and pemoline on paired-associate learning and spelling in hyperactive children." *Journal of Consulting and Clinical Psychology*. 1984, 52, 104–113.

92. Richardson, E., Kupietz, S. S., Winsberg, B. G., Maitinsky, S., and N. Mendell. "Effects of methylphenidate dosage in hyperactive reading-disabled children: II. Reading achievement." *Journal of the American Academy of Child and Adolescent Psychiatry*. 1988, 27, 78–87.

93. DuPaul, G. J., Anastopoulos, A. D., Kwasnik, D., Barkley, R. A., and M. B. McMurray. "Methylphenidate effects on children with Attention-Deficit/

Hyperactivity disorder: Self-report of symptoms, side-effects, and self-esteem." *Journal of Attention Disorders*. 1996, 1, 3–15.

94. Douglas, V. I., Barr, R. G., Desilets, J., and E. Sherman. "Do high doses of stimulants impair flexible thinking in Attention-Deficit/Hyperactivity disorder?" *Journal of the American Academy of Child and Adolescent Psychiatry*. 1995, 34, 877–885.

95. Zeiner, P. "Body growth and cardiovascular function after extended treatment (1.75 years) with methylphenidate in boys with Attention-Deficit/Hyperactivity Disorder." *Journal of Child and Adolescent Psychopharmacology*. 5, 129–138.

96. Rapport, M. D., and C. Denney. "Titrating methylphenidate in children with Attention-Deficit/Hyperactivity Disorder: Is body mass predictive of clinical response?" *Journal of the American Academy of Child and Adolescent Psychiatry*. 1997, 36, 523–530.

97. DuPaul, G. J., Anastopoulos, A. D., Kwasnik, D., Barkley, R. A., and M. B. McMurray. "Methylphenidate effects on children with Attention-Deficit/Hyperactivity disorder: Self-report of symptoms, side-effects, and self-esteem." *Journal of Attention Disorders*. 1996, 1, 3–15.

98. Weinberg, H. A. "Generic bioequivalence." (Letter to editor.) *Journal of the American Academy of Child and Adolescent Psychiatry*. 1995, 34, 834–835.

99. Safer, D. J., and R. P. Allen. "Absence of tolerance to the behavioral effects of methylphenidate in hyperactive and inattentive children." *Journal of Pediatrics*. 1989, 115, 1003–1008.

100. Connor, D. "Questions and Answers," (column). *ADHD Report*. 1995, 3, 12–13.

101. Richters, J. E., Arnold, L. E., Jensen, P. S., Abikoff, H., Conners, C. K., Greenhill, L. L., Hechtman, L., Hinshaw, S. P., Pelham, W. E., and J. M. Swanson. "NIMH collaborative multisite multimodal treatment study of children with ADHD: I. Background and rationale." *Journal of the American Academy of Child and Adolescent Psychiatry*. 1995, 34, 987–1000.

102. Volkow, N. D., Ding, Y.-S., Fowler, J. S., Wang, G.-J., Logan, J., Gatley, J. S., Dewey, S., Ashby, C., Lieberman, J., Hitzemann, R., and A. P. Wolf. "Is methylphenidate like cocaine? Studies on their pharmacokinetics and distribution in the human brain." *Archives of General Psychiatry*. 1995, 52, 456–463.

103. Spencer, T. J., Biederman, J., Harding, M., O'Donnell, D., Faraone, S. V., and T. E. Wilens. "Growth deficits in ADHD children revisited: Evidence for disorder-associated growth delays?" *Journal of the American Academy of Child and Adolescent Psychiatry*. 1996, 35, 1460–1469.

104. Spencer, T., Wilens, T., Biederman, J., Faraone, S. V., Ablon, J. S., and K. Lapey. "A double-blind, crossover comparison of methylphenidate and placebo in adults with childhood-onset Attention-Deficit/Hyperactivity Disorder." *Archives of General Psychiatry*. 1995, 52, 434–443.

105. Gadow, K. D., Sverd, J., Sprafkin, J., Nolan, E. E., and S. N. Ezor. "Efficacy of methylphenidate for Attention-Deficit/Hyperactivity Disorder in children with tic disorder. *Archives of General Psychiatry*. 1995, 52, 444–455.

106. Riddle, M. A., Lynch, K. A., Scahill, L., de Vries, A., Cohen, D. J., and J. F. Leckman. "Methylphenidate discontinuation and reinitiation during long-term treatment of children with Tourette's disorder and Attention-Deficit/Hyperactivity Disorder: A pilot study." *Journal of Child and Adolescent Psychopharmacology*. 1995, 5, 205–214.

107. Pliszka, S. R. "Effect of anxiety on cognition, behavior, and stimulant response in ADHD." *Journal of the American Academy of Child and Adolescent Psychiatry*. 1989, 28, 882–887.

108. DuPaul, G. J., Barkley, R. A., and M. B. McMurray. "Response of children with ADHD to methylphenidate: Interaction with internalizing symptoms." *Journal of the American Academy of Child and Adolescent Psychiatry*. 1994, 33, 894–903.

109. Spencer, T., Biederman, J., Wilens, T., Harding, M., O'Donnell, D., and S. Griffin. "Pharmacotherapy of Attention-Deficit/Hyperactivity Disorder across the life cycle." *Journal of the American Academy of Child and Adolescent Psychiatry*. 1996, 35, 409–432.

110. Gammon, G. D., and T. E. Brown. "Fluoxetine and methylphenidate in combination for treatment of attention deficit disorder and comorbid depressive disorder." *Journal of Child and Adolescent Psychopharmacology*. 1993, 3, 1–10.

111. Janicak, P. G., Davis, J. M., Preskorn, S. H., and F. J. Ayd. *Principles and Practice of Pharmacotherapy*. Baltimore: Williams and Wilkins, 1993, p. 281.

112. Barrickman, L. L., Perry, P. J., Allen, A. J., Kuperman, S., Arndt, S. V., Herrmann, K. J., and E. Schumacher. "Buproprion versus methylphenidate in the treatment of Attention-Deficit/Hyperactivity Disorder." *Journal of the American Academy of Child and Adolescent Psychiatry*. 1995, 34, 649–657.

113. Conners, C. K., Casat, C. D., Gualtieri, C. T., Weller, E., Reader, M., Reiss, A., Weller, R., Khayrallah, M., and J. Ascher. "Buproprion hydrochloride in Attention Deficit Disorder with Hyperactivity." *Journal of the American Academy of Child and Adolescent Psychiatry*. 1996, 35, 1314–1321.

114. Sikitch, L. "Allergic reactions to Buproprion in child psychiatric patients." *Child and Adolescent Psychopharmacology News*. 1996, 1, 1, 7.

115. Hedges, D., Reimherr, F. W., Rogers, A., Strong, R., and P. H.

Wender. "An open trial of venlafaxine in adult patients with Attention Deficit Hyperactivity Disorder." *Psychopharmacology Bulletin.* 1995, 31, 779–783.

116. Adler, L. A., Resnick, S., Junz, M., and O. Devinsky. Open-label trial of venlafaxine in adults with Attention Deficit Disorder. *Psychopharmacology Bulletin.* 1995, 31, 785–788.

117. Hornig-Rohan, M., and J. D. Amsterdam. "Venlafaxine versus stimulant therapy in patients with dual diagnoses of Attention-Deficit Disorder and depression." *Psychopharmacology Bulletin.* 1995, 31, 580.

118. Olvera, R. L., Pliszka, S. R., Luh, J., and R. Tatum. "An open trial of venlafaxine in the treatment of Attention-Deficit/Hyperactivity Disorder in children and adolescents." *Journal of Child and Adolescent Psychopharmacology.* 1996, 6, 241–250.

119. Hunt, R. D., Minderaa, R. B., and D. J. Cohen. "Clonidine benefits children with attention deficit disorder and hyperactivity: Report of a double-blind placebo-controlled crossover study." *Journal of the American Academy of Child Psychiatry.* 1985, 24, 617–629.

120. Leckman, J. F., Hardin, M. T., Riddle, M. A., Stevenson, J., Ort, S., and D. J. Cohen. "Clonidine treatment of Gilles de la Tourette's syndrome." *Archives of General Psychiatry.* 1991, 48, 324–328.

121. Hunt, R. D., Capper, L., and P. O'Connell. "Clonidine in childhood and adolescent psychiatry." *Journal of Child and Adolescent Psychopharmacology.* 1990, 1, 87–102.

122. Wilens, T. E., Biederman, J., and T. Spencer. "Clonidine for sleep disturbances associated with Attention-Deficit/Hyperactivity Disorder." *Journal of the American Academy of Child and Adolescent Psychiatry.* 1994, 33, 424–426.

123. Horacek, H. J. "Extended-release clonidine for sleep disorders." (Letter to the editor.) *Journal of the American Academy of Child and Adolescent Psychiatry.* 1994, 33, 1210.

124. Dulcan, M. K. "The safe and effective use of psychotropic medications in adolescents and children: Information for parents and youth on psychotropic medications." *Journal of Child and Adolescent Psychopharmacology.* 1992, 2, 81–101.

125. Hunt, R. D., Arnsten, A.F.T., and M. D. Asbell. "An open trial of guanfacine in the treatment of Attention-Deficit/Hyperactivity Disorder." *Journal of the American Academy of Child and Adolescent Psychiatry.* 1995, 34, 50–54.

126. Chappell, P. B., Riddle, M. A., Scahill, L., Lynch, K. A., Schultz, R., Arnsten, A., Leckman, J. F., and D. J. Cohen. "Guanfacine treatment of comorbid Attention-Deficit/Hyperactivity Disorder and Tourette's Syndrome: Preliminary clinical experience." *Journal of the American Academy of Child and Adolescent Psychiatry.* 1995, 34, 1140–1146.

127. Wilens, T. E., Spencer, T., Biederman, J., Wozniak, J., and D. Connor. "Combined pharmacotherapy: An emerging trend in pediatric psychopharmacology." *Journal of the American Academy of Child and Adolescent Psychiatry.* 1995, 34, 110–112.

128. Bastiaens, L. "The impact of an intensive educational program on knowledge, attitudes, and side effects of psychotropic medications among adolescent inpatients." *Journal of Child and Adolescent Psychopharmacology.* 1992, 2, 249–258.

129. Rosenthal, N. E. *Winter Blues: Seasonal Affective Disorder—What It Is and How to Overcome It.* New York: Guilford Press, 1993, p. 155.

130. "Mental health: does therapy help?" *Consumer Reports.* November 1995, 734–739.

131. Target, M., and P. Fonagy. "The efficacy of psychoanalysis for children with emotional disorders." *Journal of the American Academy of Child and Adolescent Psychiatry.* 1994, 33, 361–371.

132. Brown, R. T., Wynne, M. E., and R. Medenis. "Methylphenidate and cognitive therapy: A comparison of treatment approaches with hyperactive boys." *Journal of Abnormal Child Psychology.* 1985, 13, 69–87.

133. Abikoff, H., and R. Gittelman. "Hyperactive children treated with stimulants." *Archives of General Psychiatry.* 1985, 42, 953–961.

134. Ellis, A. *Reason and Emotion in Psychotherapy.* New York: Lyle Stuart, 1962.

135. Lewinsohn, P. M., Hoberman, H. M., and G. N. Clarke. "The Coping with Depression Course: Review and future directions." *Canadian Journal of Behavioral Science.* 1989, 21, 470–493.

136. Markus, E., Lange, A., and T. F. Pettigrew. "Effectiveness of family therapy: A meta analysis." *Journal of Family Therapy.* 1990, 12, 205–221.

137. Alexander, J. F., and B. V. Parsons. *Functional Family Therapy.* Monterey, Cal.: Brooks/Cole, 1982, p. 73.

138. Wachtel, E. F. *Treating Troubled Children and Their Families.* New York: Guilford Press, 1994, p. 3.

139. Barkley, R. A. *Defiant Children: A Clinician's Manual for Parent Training.* New York: Guilford Press, 1987.

140. Phelan, T. W. *1-2-3 Magic: Training Your Preschooler and Preteen to Do What You Want.* Glen Ellyn, Ill.: Child Management Inc., 1984, passim.

141. Picchietti, D. L., and A. S. Walters. "Restless legs syndrome and periodic limb movement disorder in children and adolescents: Comorbidity with Attention-Deficit/Hyperactivity Disorder." In Dahl, R. E., ed. *Child and Adolescent Psychiatric Clinics of North America.* 1996, 5, 729–740.

142. Gaultier, C. "Clinical and therapeutic aspects of obstructive sleep apnea syndrome in infants and children." *Sleep*. 1992 Supplement, 36–38.

143. Dahl, R. E. "Sleep in behavioral and emotional disorders." In Ferber, R., and Kryger, M., eds. *Principles and Practice of Sleep Medicine in the Child*. Philadelphia: W. B. Saunders, 1995, 147–154.

144. Dahlitz, M., Alvarez, B., Vignau, J., English, J., Arendt, J., and J. D. Parkes. "Delayed sleep phase response to melatonin." *Lancet*. 1991, 337, 1121–1124.

145. Jan, J. E., Espezel, H., and R. E. Appleton. "The treatment of sleep disorders with melatonin." *Developmental Medicine and Child Neurology*. 1994, 36, 97–107.

146. Biederman, J., Santangelo, S. L., Faraone, S. V., Kiely, K., Guite, J., Mick, E., Reed, E. D., Kraus, I., Jollinek, J., and J. Perrin. "Clinical correlates of enuresis in ADHD and non-ADHD children." *Journal of Child Psychology and Psychiatry*. 1995, 36, 865–877.

147. Barclay, D. R., and A. C. Houts. "Childhood enuresis." In Schaefer, C. E., ed. *Clinical Handbook of Sleep Disorders in Children*. Northvale, N.J.: Jason Aronson, 1995, pp. 223–252.

148. Sheldon, S. H. "Sleep-related enuresis." *Child and Adolescent Psychiatric Clinics of North America*. 1996, 661–672.

149. Fritz, G. K., Rockney, R. M., and A. S. Yeung. "Plasma levels and efficacy of imipramine treatment for enuresis." *Journal of the American Academy of Child and Adolescent Psychiatry*. 1994, 33, 60–64.

150. Thompson, S., and J. M. Rey. "Functional enuresis: Is desmopressin the answer?" *Journal of the American Academy of Child and Adolescent Psychiatry*. 1995, 34, 266–271.

151. Price, J. M., and K. A. Dodge. "Peers' contributions to children's social maladjustment: Description and intervention." In Berndt, T. J., and G. W. Ladd, eds. *Peer Relationships in Child Development*. New York: John Wiley, 1989, pp. 341–370.

152. Olson, S. L. "Development of conduct problems and peer rejection in preschool children: A social systems analysis." *Journal of Abnormal Child Psychology*. 1992, 20, 327–350.

153. Barkley, R. A. *Taking Charge of ADHD*. New York: Guilford Press, 1995, p. 3.

154. Phelan, T. *1-2-3 Magic: Training Your Preschoolers and Preteens to Do What You Want*. Glen Ellyn, Ill.: Child Management, Inc., 1984, p. 3.

155. Reid, M. J., O'Leary, S. G., and L. S. Wolff. "Effects of maternal distraction and reprimands on toddlers' transgressions and negative affect." *Journal of Abnormal Child Psychology*. 1994, 22, 237–245.

156. Acker, M. M., and S. G. O'Leary. "Inconsistency of mothers' feedback and toddlers' misbehavior and negative affect." *Journal of Abnormal Child Psychology.* 1996, 24, 703–714.

157. Straus, M. A., Gelles, R. J., and S. K. Steinmetz. *Behind Closed Doors: Violence in the American Family.* New York: Anchor Press/Doubleday, 1980, passim.

158. Ingersoll, B. D. "Psychiatric disorders among adopted children: a review and commentary." *Adoption Quarterly.* in press.

159. Allen, R. "When adoption and learning/attention difficulties overlap: The impact on the adoptive family." Unpublished manuscript. The Barker Foundation, 1996.

160. Kelly, K., and P. Ramundo. *You Mean I'm Not Lazy, Stupid or Crazy?!* Cincinnati, Oh.: Tyrell & Jerem Press, 1993, passim.

161. Hallowell, E. M., and J. J. Ratey. *Driven to Distraction.* New York: Pantheon, 1994, passim.

162. Nadeau, K. G., ed. *A Comprehensive Guide to Attention Deficit Disorder in Adults.* New York: Brunner/Mazel, 1995.

163. Wender, P. H. *Attention-Deficit Hyperactivity Disorder in Adults.* New York: Oxford University Press, 1995, p. 29.

164. Tannen, D. *You Just Don't Understand.* New York: William Morrow, 1990, p. 143.

165. Beach, S.R.H., Sandeen, E. E., and E. D. O'Leary. *Depression in Marriage.* New York: Guilford Press, 1990, p. 62.

166. Kahn, J., Coyne, J. C., and G. Margolin. "Depression and Marital Conflict: The Social Construction of Despair." *Journal of Social and Personal Relationships.* 1985, 2, 447–462.

167. Rohrkemper, M. "Individual Differences in Students' Perceptions of Routine Classroom Events." *Journal of Educational Psychology.* 1985, 77, 29–44.

168. Stoner, G., and S. K. Green. "A pilot study of instruction in and understanding of classroom rules in the primary grades." Unpublished manuscript cited in G. J. DuPaul and G. Stoner, eds. *ADHD in the Schools: Assessment and Intervention Strategies.* New York: Guilford Press, 1994, p. 124.

169. Pfiffner, L. J., and S. G. O'Leary. "The efficacy of all-positive management as a function of the prior use of negative consequences." *Journal of Applied Behavior Analysis.* 1987, 20, 265–271.

170. Zentall, S. "Modifying classroom tasks and environments." In S. Goldstein, ed. *Understanding and Managing Children's Classroom Behavior.* New York: John Wiley, 1995, pp. 356–374.

171. Barclay, J. R. "Effecting behavior change in the elementary classroom: An exploratory study." *Journal of Counseling Psychology*. 1967, 14, 240–247.

172. Hatcher, P. J., Hulme, C., and A. W. Ellis. "Ameliorating early reading failure by integrating the teaching of reading and phonological skills: The phonological linkage hypothesis." *Child Development*. 1994, 65, 41–57.

173. Kearney, C. A., and R. S. Drabman. "The write-say method for improving spelling accuracy in children with learning disabilities." *Journal of Learning Disabilities*. 1993, 26, 52–56.

174. Swanson, J. M., Kotkin, R., Pfiffner, L., and K. McBurnett. "School-Based Interventions for ADHD Students." *CH.A.D.D.ER*. 1992, 6, 8–9, 22.

175. Swanson, J. M. "ADD research: A look at today and tomorrow." An interview with Russell A. Barkley, Ph.D. *Attention*. 1996, 3, 1, 9–11.

176. Swanson, J. M. "ADD research: A look at today and tomorrow." An interview with Peter S. Jensen, M.D. *Attention*. 1996, 3, 1, 11–14.

177. Quinn, P. O. "Neurobiology of Attention Deficit Disorder." In K. G. Nadeau, ed. *A Comprehensive Guide to Attention Deficit Disorder in Adults: Research, Diagnosis, and Treatment*. New York: Brunner/Mazel, 1995, pp. 18–31.

178. Eist, H. I. "Response to the presidential address: Why we must prevail." *American Journal of Psychiatry*. 1996, 153, 1123–1125.

INDEX

Index

233